Elsebeth Stenager, MD, PhD
Egon Stenager, MD

Disease, Pain,
and Suicidal Behavior

Pre-publication
REVIEWS,
COMMENTARIES,
EVALUATIONS . . .

"**A**n encyclopedic review of the epidemiology of suicide in disease. Recommended to all medical professionals who are faced with suicide or suicidal behavior and chronic disease, be they psychiatrists, neurologists, internists, social workers, or health care authorities, but first and foremost researchers in epidemiology of suicidal behavior. The message of the book is that many suicides could be prevented if patients were given proper care and the victims' warning signals were appropriately interpreted. Although the approach is purely scientific, it never becomes academic in the negative sense, and the care for suffering and distressed fellow human beings, although unspoken, goes through the book as a red thread."

Nils Koch-Henriksen, MD, DMSc
Director, Danish Multiple Sclerosis Registry, Alborg, Denmark

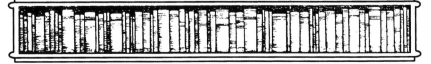

More pre-publication
REVIEWS, COMMENTARIES, EVALUATIONS . . .

"**T**his book highlights the fact
that suicidal behavior is a
phenomenon found in patients in
most medical specialties and not
only psychiatry. . . . It will stimu-
late people working in health care
to widen their perspectives and ini-
tiate interdisciplinary dialogues–all
hopefully resulting in a better
understanding of the problem of
suicide."

Lil Träskman-Bendz, MD, PhD
Professor of Psychiatry
Department of Clinical Neuroscience
University Hospital
Lund, Sweden

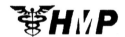

The Haworth Medical Press
An Imprint of The Haworth Press, Inc.

Disease, Pain, and Suicidal Behavior

THE HAWORTH MEDICAL PRESS
New, Recent, and Forthcoming Titles
of Related Interest

Disease, Pain, and Suicidal Behavior

Elsebeth Nylev Stenager, MD, PhD
Egon Stenager, MD

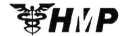

The Haworth Medical Press
An Imprint of The Haworth Press, Inc.
New York • London

Published by

The Haworth Medical Press, Inc., an imprint of The Haworth Press, Inc., 10 Alice Street, Binghamton, NY 13904-1580

DISCLAIMER

Medicine is an ever-changing science. As new research and clinical experience broaden our knowledge, changes in treatment and drug therapy are required. While many suggestions for drug usages are made herein, the book is intended for educational purposes only, and the author, editor, and publisher do not accept liability in the event of negative consequences incurred as a result of information presented in this book. We do not claim that this information is necessarily accurate by the rigid, scientific standard applied for medical proof, and therefore make no warranty, expressed or implied, with respect to the material herein contained. Therefore the patient is urged to consult his or her own physician prior to following a course of treatment. The physician is urged to check the product information sheet included in the package of each drug he or she plans to administer to be certain the protocol followed is not in conflict with the manufacturer's inserts. When a discrepancy arises between these inserts and information in this book, the physician is encouraged to use his or her best professional judgement.

Cover design by Monica L. Seifert.

Library of Congress Cataloging-in-Publication Data

Stenager, Elsebeth.
    Disease, pain, and suicidal behavior / Elsebeth Nylev Stenager, Egon Stenager.
        p.   cm.
    Includes bibliographical references and index.
    ISBN 0-7890-0295-7 (alk. paper).
    1. Suicidal behavior. 2. Psychological manifestations of general diseases. I. Stenager, Egon. II. Title.
RC569.S82   1997
616.85′8445–dc21   97-15308
                                                                       CIP

To Kirstina, Maria, Søren, and Jacob

ABOUT THE AUTHORS

Elsebeth Nylev Stenager, MD, PhD, is Senior Public Health Physician in the Department of Social Medicine at Odense Municipality in Odense, Denmark. For the last ten years, her research has focused on suicidal behavior and somatic disorders. A member of the Danish section of the WHO/Euro Multicenter Study on Parasuicide, she used the results of this study as the foundation for her PhD thesis *Attempted Suicide, Treatment and Outcome.* Dr. Stenager is the author of many articles and abstracts as well as a frequent lecturer.

Egon Stenager, MD, is Senior Neurological Consultant in the Department of Neurology at Esbjerg Hospital in Esbjerg, Denmark. A co-founder of the Neuropsychiatric Research Unit and a former Associate Professor in the Department of Neurology at Odense University Hospital, he is presently a consultant at the Danish Multiple Sclerosis Registry in Copenhagen. The author of more than sixty papers and a co-editor of several books and periodicals, Dr. Stenager has given numerous lectures in several countries. A great deal of his research has focused on neurological disorders, with special emphasis on behavioral and neuropsychiatric aspects of neurology.

CONTENTS

Foreword

In daily work in the health sector, all professionals use much of their time treating, helping, and counseling patients with chronic diseases. This can be very difficult, as patients often suffer from severe, intractable pain for which there is no relief. The psychological factor can often be an essential part of pain, but in any case, it can create severe problems for doctors, nurses, and other health care professionals.

For the therapeutic team, it is often surprising that severely chronically ill patients, often even though they suffer from severe pain, wish to go on living. Some commit suicide, and some attempt suicide. In some cases, the suicidal behavior can be explained by the very unhappy patient's need to draw attention to his or her problems.

But how can therapeutic teams within or outside hospital regimen help the patient find quality in life in spite of a hopeless condition that, in the eyes of others, could justify suicide?

Both Elsebeth and Egon Stenager have worked for a long period of time in the Department of Psychiatry, Odense University Hospital in Denmark, during which I was their supervisor. When the department joined the WHO European Project on Suicidal Behavior, Elsebeth Stenager conducted a substudy in the project on the County of Funen, Denmark. The results were presented as a monograph for which she was awarded her doctorate at Odense University.

Her husband, Egon Stenager, and I worked together for a number of years on multiple sclerosis and our studies especially concentrated on the cognitive deficits occurring in those with the disease. Although at the time the aspect was not recognized as very important, we published a number of articles in which we clearly illustrated the significance of cognitive deficits caused by multiple sclerosis. During our studies, we learned a great deal about life quality for patients suffering from chronic diseases. This resulted in the presentation of papers on pain associated with multiple sclerosis.

Through our work, both with patients with suicidal behavior and with patients with multiple sclerosis, we very soon found that there was a tremendous need for counseling, for support, for advice, and for professional help for these patients. We suddenly realized that this dimension was also a subject that should be researched in projects on suicidal behavior and multiple sclerosis. We met patients who asked clearly whether life was worth living in their condition. At the same time, we also experienced that even in very hopeless conditions, patients often cling to life. It was then natural to conclude that there was a need to examine both the patients' reasons for trying to commit suicide, and also the reason why others wished to go on living even when their condition was considered hopeless by others. Where did they find reasonable quality of life?

In the authors, this gave rise to the idea to compile the present book, as they were aware of the need among professionals in the health sector to learn how they could best support their patients through this difficult stage in life. Good counseling, good professional support, and a humane attitude is needed when getting close to hopelessly ill patients, some of them suffering from severe pain. It is important to have a knowledge of the mechanisms behind their mental reactions and also to find a way to be a kind, humane professional without lapsing into useless sentimentality.

In this book you will not find answers to all these questions, but you will find a description of the experience of two specialists in the field.

Knud Jensen, MD
Chief Psychiatrist and Neurologist
Department of Psychiatry
Odense University Hospital
Denmark

Chapter 1

General Aspects
of Suicidal Behavior

Suicides and suicide attempts are very frequent incidents in the Western hemisphere. Buzan and Weissberg (1992) estimate that in 1988, in the United States 30,407 deaths were due to suicide. This figure indicates that every eighth death in the United States is due to suicide, and every third death among those aged fifteen to twenty-four years is caused by suicide.

For years the suicide rate in the United States constantly has been 12.5 suicides per 100,000 persons per year. However, the frequency of suicide has increased among young people, whereas it has decreased among the elderly. An increased suicide rate has also occurred among young black men. Thus, the frequency of suicide is now similar in young black and young Caucasian men. However, in general the frequency of suicide among blacks is 50 percent higher than in the Caucasian population. Furthermore, the mortality rate is higher among blacks due to homicide.

The research on mortality rates in other ethnic minorities in the United States has been minimal. Though, in general other ethnic minorities have a lower mortality rate to suicide compared to Caucasians. The mortality due to suicide in men is higher than in women, with a ratio of 3:1 to 4:1. The methods most frequently used are shooting, hanging, strangling, and poisoning with medication.

Especially among the young, a dramatic increase in the frequency of suicide has been seen within the last four decades. In certain areas, it has almost been like an epidemic. An increase from 4 per 100,000 per year in 1950 to 13.2 per 100,000 per year in 1988 in the fifteen- to twenty-four-year-old age group has been found. This increase has been seen not just in the United States, but also in a number of European countries.

However, the number of actual suicides is just the tip of the iceberg. It has been estimated that the number of suicide attempts is at least eight to ten times the number of suicides. Furthermore, the number of suicides probably is underestimated and uncertain due to methodological problems concerning registering suicides. Monk (1987) has described several factors contributing to this underregistration.

In the United States, information on mortality due to suicide is collected in each state separately. Consequently, geographic considerations, cultural influences, and varying time periods for the studies can cause great variation in which cases deaths are registered as suicide.

In order to be sure that a death is due to suicide, ideally, it is necessary to perform a psychological autopsy, during which close relatives, friends, and others are queried about the indicators of suicide. Such a procedure is not possible because it is time-consuming and expensive.

A further problem in the United States is that persons with various types of training fill in the death certificates, and thereby decide the cause of death. No doubt, a medically trained person in cooperation with a forensic pathologist would be the most appropriate person to determine the cause of death as he or she would not be influenced by political or social pressure, and thus would not omit suicide as a cause of death. Additionally, a medically trained person is expected to register more suicides than, for example, a sheriff or mortician. Due to these factors, the validity of suicide statistics in the United States has to be taken with considerable reservation. These problems also have to be taken into account when reading the next chapters on methodological problems.

The frequency of suicide in Europe does not differ much from that of the United States. An increasing frequency of suicide has also been seen in Europe within the last few decades. This caused the World Health Organization (WHO) in *Target for Health for All: The health policy for Europe* in 1985 to adopt as their twelfth goal:

> By the year 2000, there should be a sustained and continuing reduction in the prevalence of mental disorders, an improvement in the quality of life of all people with such disorders, and a reversal of the rising trends in suicide and attempted suicide.

At the same time, a large common European Project was planned, in which suicide attempts in certain representative areas in several European countries were registered, and interviews with representative suicide attempters were performed (Bille-Brahe, 1993; Stenager, 1996). One of the purposes of the project was to identify risk factors for suicide and repetitive suicide attempts in a high-risk group such as suicide attempters. The suicide rates in different countries varied. In former Communist countries, such as Hungary, the frequency of suicide was 44 per 100,000 per year. Countries such as Finland, Denmark, Germany, France, Austria, and Switzerland also had high suicide rates, with rates above 20 per 100,000 per year. The lowest rates, comparable to the level in the United States, were found in Sweden, Norway, and the Netherlands.

Based on the common European registration study, it also has been possible to estimate the frequency of suicide attempts in the involved areas. The number of suicide attempts is low in the Netherlands and Italy while Finland, England, and Denmark have suicide attempt rates of 200 to 300 per 100,000 per year (Bille-Brahe, 1993).

The primary goal in the research of risk factors in suicides and suicide attempts has been to reveal social and psychiatric characteristics in suicidal persons. Research has revealed that a number of psychiatric disorders such as depression, schizophrenia, personality disorders, anxiety disorders, and abuse of alcohol and drugs are risk factors for suicidal behavior.

Furthermore, a large number of social factors are thought to be of importance in suicidal behavior, such as recent divorce or dependence on public support, for example, financial support for the unemployed or welfare. Variation due to gender is also found. The risk of suicide is higher among men than women, while the frequency of suicide attempts is higher among women than men. Older people more frequently commit suicide than younger people, while younger people more frequently attempt suicide than older people.

Beyond the social and psychiatric factors, research groups also have examined the association between suicidal behavior and biological factors (Roy, DeJong, Linnoila, 1989). Träskman and colleagues (1992) examined the content of the metabolites 5-hydroxyindoleacetic acid (HIAA), homovanilin acid, and 3-methoxy 4-hydroxyphenylglycol in the cerebrospinal fluid of patients who had made suicide attempts. They found an association between a low level of HIAA and certain types of suicide attempts. Patients who made violent suicide attempts had a low level of HIAA. Other researchers have found the same association; however, all the studies are based on small populations. Therefore, final conclusions on the association of biological markers and suicidal behavior are not yet possible.

In connection with the prevention of suicide and the treatment of patients who have made suicide attempts, it is important to be able to predict which groups are at risk of either committing suicide or repeating a suicide attempt. A lot of suicide-threatened persons contact their practitioner or other health or social work personnel in the weeks or months just before they make their suicide attempt or commit suicide (Stenager and Jensen, 1994). However, if the warning signals or risk factors are not known and recognized, the chance of prevention is really small.

Within recent decades, several studies have been performed in order to identify risk factors. The studies have concentrated on social and psychiatric characteristics of suicidal persons. Despite this vast number of studies, almost none have dealt with the association of physical disorders and suicidal behavior. A reason may be that suicidal behavior in many countries is considered to be a psychiatric problem, and therefore, such behavior rarely catches the attention of somatically interested doctors—neither from the point of view of research nor treatment.

Neurological disorders and cancer are the only sufferings in which suicidal behavior has been studied carefully. Such studies have been of fair quality, judged from a methodological point of view. As a contrast, studies on much more frequent somatic disorders and suicidal behavior usually are either nonexistent or outdated and inconclusive due to methodological flaws.

Some Danish studies (Nielsen, Wang, and Bille-Brahe, 1990; Nielsen, 1994; Stenager and Benjaminsen, 1991) have been performed specifically in order to understand the importance of somatic disorders as risk factors in suicide attempts, but the number is few.

From the point of view of both prevention and treatment, it would be of utmost importance if not only health personal in psychiatric wards but also health personnel in somatic wards were aware of both general risk factors for suicidal behavior and somatic disorders associated with an increased risk of suicide. Using this knowledge, such personnel could establish a better psychosocial treatment of the endangered groups of patients, thereby increasing their quality of life while decreasing the acknowledged increased risk of suicidal behavior.

Suicidal behavior could be regarded as the ultimate consequence of a life that for a number of reasons is unbearable. Therefore, in certain cases, the circumstances will be such that no treatment can be expected to be helpful, and prevention may be difficult or even impossible. Consequently, not all suicides can be prevented. However, a large number of physical, psychological, medical, and psychosocial conditions can be changed, which may alleviate the life of a severely strained person, and thus with proper treatment and support, make the life bearable. Then, the question is whether we today have the necessary knowledge and resources to provide this help, especially to patients with chronic somatic disorders.

The purpose of this book is to give a review of the psychosocial problems associated with a chronic somatic disorder, methodological problems in suicide research especially regarding somatic disorders and suicidal behavior, and our present knowledge on the association of specific somatic disorders, pains, and suicidal behavior. Finally, based on this review, proposals for prevention and treatment of this group of patients will be presented.

Chapter 2

Psychosocial Aspects
of Chronic Somatic Disorders

Traditionally, the task of doctors has been to diagnose and treat disorders, while the more delicate problems of how a disorder affects the patient and his or her surroundings have either been neglected or dealt with by relatives, nurses, social workers, and others. Consequently, almost nothing can be found in medical literature on this aspect. However, in the context of suicide and chronic somatic disorders, the effects of a disorder are important in order to understand why people with, for example, a neurological disorder may have an increased risk of suicide. Therefore, in this chapter the present knowledge on the psychosocial aspect of one neurological disorder, i.e., multiple sclerosis, is presented.

Some of the findings are unique to multiple sclerosis, but most are common not only in dealing with neurological disorders but also with other disorders.

Multiple sclerosis is fully described in Chapter 5. Here, however, only disease courses and prognosis are mentioned, which is intended to give a basis for understanding the following descriptions.

COURSE AND PROGNOSIS

An important concept in multiple sclerosis is an attack or relapse, which means a usually transient deterioration, i.e., an outbreak of the disorder. This could be a paralysis, sensory disturbances, visual disturbances, or other problems lasting from a few days up to several months. A remission, i.e., a disappearance of the symptoms, may then occur. A new relapse may or may not happen again in the future with varying intervals of time between such attacks.

The course of the disease can be described in different ways, but the following terms are often used.

1. *Relapsing/remitting course.* The course is characterized by repeating relapses and remissions, usually lasting weeks to months. At the onset, the relapses often occur frequently. Later on the course may change to a secondary progressive course.
2. *The secondary progressive course.* This course is characterized by a gradual, and usually slow, deterioration with no remissions.
3. *The primary progressive course.* The deterioration occurs gradually from the onset with no remission.
4. *Benign multiple sclerosis.* Only few relapses are seen and the symptoms are mild. (Confavreux, Aimard, and Devic, 1980; Weinshenker et al., 1989; Thompson et al., 1990)

The onset of multiple sclerosis may be acute, so that a stroke or brain tumor is suspected, but usually a long period passes from the time the first symptom occurs until the diagnosis is made (Stenager and Jensen, 1993). The period from onset to diagnosis is frequently five to six years (Confavreux, Aimard, and Devic, 1980; Stenager, Knudsen, and Jensen, 1989). New diagnostic procedures may reduce this period in the years to come. At the time of diagnosis, roughly 20 percent of the patients have a primary progressive course.

Patients with a relapsing/remitting course who progress to a secondary progressive course will on the average do so after approximately seven years. Expressed differently, ten to twelve years after diagnosis, 40 to 50 percent of patients with relapsing/remitting course will have changed to a secondary progressive course (Confavreux, Aimard, and Devic, 1980; Weinshenker et al., 1989; Lauer and Firnhaber, 1987).

Prognosis can be measured in different ways. In this context a very simplistic model will be used: slight, moderate, and severe impairment. A slightly impaired patient will be able to take care of him- or herself without aids while a moderately impaired patient typically will use a cane, and a severely impaired patient will use a wheelchair or be bedridden.

Five years after the diagnosis has been made, approximately 25 percent will be moderately impaired and approximately 50 to 60 percent after fifteen years. Generally, 30 percent have a benign course, and 10 to 15 percent a severe course. Finally, a study found that 60 percent were alive thirty-five years after the diagnosis was made (Poser et al., 1989).

PREDIAGNOSTIC PERIOD

The prediagnostic period is defined as the period between the first symptom of multiple sclerosis and when the diagnosis is made. The patient experiences this period as a time of searching for an explanation of the symptoms and experiencing uncertainty. This is reflected by the fact that approximately 10 percent of the patients are admitted to a psychiatric ward in this period, and a further 10 percent have their symptoms of multiple sclerosis misinterpreted as a surgical disorder (Stenager and Jensen, 1988; 1993).

Relatives also find this period characterized by uncertainty, due to both anxiety regarding the cause of the symptoms and doubt over whether the patient suffers from a somatic or a psychiatric disorder. Finally, the family physician also may be uncertain of the nature of the symptoms.

This period may last for years (Marteux, 1991; Burnfield and Burnfield, 1978, 1982; Duval, 1984).

THE DIAGNOSTIC PERIOD

Obviously, the diagnostic period is associated with much anxiety both for the patient and relatives due to fear of what diagnosis may be reached, treatment possibilities, and prognosis. The treating physician may have doubts regarding how to inform the patient and relatives and how much is to be told. Frequently, little or nothing is told (Stenager, Knudsen, and Jensen, 1989; Burnfield, 1984; Elian and Dean, 1985; Spencer, 1988; Stewart and Sullivans, 1982).

Some of the patients will experience a crisis reaction. Of course, this can also occur at other stages of the disorder, such as a relapse or transition to a secondary progressive course.

CRISIS REACTION

The first stage in the crisis reaction is the *denial*. In denial, the patient refuses to accept the diagnosis. He will consult other authorities in order to have the diagnosis rejected. He will not meet other patients with multiple sclerosis, and he will try to hide the diagnosis. Trying to maintain previous activities and refusing to accept help from others also characterize this stage of behavior.

The next stage is the *resistance phase*, in which the patient anxiously seeks information on multiple sclerosis and tries to control the disease. Reluctantly, he will accept help from others. He may accept meeting other patients with multiple sclerosis and perhaps participate in self-help groups.

The third stage is *acceptance*. The patient now confronts the disease and starts to redefine activities and life qualities. He feels sorry for loss of previous independence and openly acknowledges the disease. He learns to accept help from others and redefines the meaning of a chronic disorder and impairment.

The final phase is *integration*, which requires a long period until it is reached. The patient will face new problems associated with the disorder with a minimum use of emotional energy and will have the power to deal with other things than his own disease. He will find certain advantages in the present situation, allow others to help him, and express gratitude for the help received.

POSTDIAGNOSTIC PERIOD

The length of the postdiagnostic period usually is long, and the course will depend on the course of the disease. Psychosocial aspects in different courses of the disease have not been studied. The following is based on a few cross-sectional studies and one follow-up study and will deal with self-esteem, demographic factors, social and leisure activities, habitation, economy, and the need for help.

Matson and Brooks (1989) have made a questionnaire study on psychosocial adjustment in 174 patients with multiple sclerosis, equivalent of 60 percent of the patients asked. The authors concluded that with increasing duration of illness, a better adjustment occurred despite increasing impairment. Adjustment occurs within the first five to ten years, and then the adaptation or integration is stable. Factors that facilitate adaptation are support from the family and support from one's religion; however, accepting the disorder and exhibiting a need to fight the disorder indicated maladaptation. Brooks and Matson (1982) also made a nine-year follow-up study of the same patients, resulting in participation of 103 patients, equivalent of approximately 60 percent of the possible participants. Based on a group estimation, the self-esteem and adjustment was almost equal at both study points, but worse than in a healthy control group. Factors that resulted in a reduced self-esteem were many symptoms, decreasing mobility, many relapses, while self-esteem was improved by high income and work capability. A gender difference was also found. Self-respect in women increased over time, and they had a more positive outlook while the opposite trend was found in men. Therefore, the authors had to revise their conclusion from the first study. Their final conclusion was that patients who accepted their disorder and fought it were doing better than patients supported by their family and religion.

A cross-sectional study by Büchi, Buddeberg, and Sieber (1989) from Switzerland found the same gender difference in an questionnaire study of 298 patients with multiple sclerosis, equivalent to 50 percent of the patients asked. Despite more somatic complaints, the women were more optimistic. This attitude improved if they were capable of working. Men were more anxious, especially if the duration of illness was short, and they tried to stay at work as long as possible.

The above-mentioned results should be estimated in the light of the previous mentioned crisis reaction, which to some extent could explain the results.

Three cross-sectional studies of 518 patients found that 70 to 75 percent of the patients were married, which corresponds to the expected percent from the background population (Brooks and Matson, 1982; Büchi, Buddeberg, and Sieber, 1989; Stenager et al., 1994). Approximately 10 to 15 percent were divorced. The risk of divorce increased with increasing impairment. In one Danish study, more men than women were divorced. Fertility does not seem to be reduced in patients with multiple sclerosis, but in some cases of divorce, patients with multiple sclerosis lose custody of their children (Stenager et al., 1994).

A Danish cross-sectional study by Stenager and colleagues (1994) of 117 patients with multiple sclerosis found that 70 percent of the patients had unchanged social activity after onset of the disorder; 25 percent lost contact with friends, and 5 percent with family. More than 80 percent had daily contact with close relatives. Outgoing activities were more difficult to maintain, as 45 percent participated in fewer activities after onset. Club-related activities were greatly reduced, and to a lesser extent, participation in cultural activities lessened. The risk of reducing activity increased with added impairment.

A study on patients' and relatives' perceptions of the social and leisure activities of the patients found a discrepancy, especially in moderately disabled patients. In this group, the patient was not as active as he reported himself to be, according to the relatives. The patient tried to maintain previous social activity on the cost of leisure activities. Women and older patients had difficulty fulfilling the expectations of the relatives. In the group with slight and severe impairment, patients and relatives agreed to a large extent. However, severely impaired patients reported more leisure activities than their relatives reported on their behalf. This discrepancy could to some extent be explained by cognitive deficits also met in this patient group. Patients who had been ill for a long period and older patients were more isolated than young patients and patients with a short duration of illness. In one Danish study, 70 percent lived in their own home, and 35 percent have had made changes so that they could stay in their home. Only the severely disabled lived in nursing homes (Stenager et al., 1994).

Two cross-sectional studies with a total of 415 patients (Büchi, Buddeberg, and Sieber, 1989; Stenager et al., 1994) showed that 60 to 70 percent received early pensions and the likelihood of receiving early pensions increased with growing impairment. A Norwegian study of 79 patients found that the characteristics of unemployed patients were onset after the age of thirty, progressive course, and hard manual work (Grønning, Hannisdal, and Mellgren, 1990). However, the financial situation differs in different societies (Confavreux, Aimard, and Devic, 1980).

Finally, the disorder affects not only the patients but also relatives. The Danish study showed that 56 percent of the patients received help from relatives, most frequently from a spouse and rarely from children. An English study found that in 70 percent of the studied population, relatives had to get up twice or more in the night to help the diseased person, and there was also need of help during the day (Spackman et al., 1989).

CONCLUSION

With multiple sclerosis as an example, this review has shown that at least three periods exist that in different ways may put strain on the patients.

In the prediagnostic period, patients have unexplained, perhaps misinterpreted, troublesome symptoms, which may lead to unexpected reactions in the patient. Obviously, the diagnostic period is associated with much anxiety and perhaps a crisis reaction. The postdiagnostic period may be even worse because expectations of treatment possibilities are not fulfilled, adaptation to a chronic disorder is difficult, the reaction of the surroundings may change, and many unexpected social consequences are taking place.

However, this situation is not unique to multiple sclerosis. The problems described in the diagnostic and postdiagnostic period can occur in any disorder, even in disorders where apparently fine treatment options exist, but where it turns out that life with a chronic disorder is more complicated than expected. Disorders with an acute and dramatic onset obviously do not have a prediagnostic period, but many disorders have such a period. Therefore, it is advised that the reader consider these three periods and their consequences when reading the following chapters on suicide and somatic disorders.

Chapter 3

Suicidal Behavior
and Mental Disorders

As previously stressed, mental disorders are of major importance as a risk factor in suicidal behavior. In contrast to somatic disorders and suicidal behavior, numerous papers have been published on mental disorders and suicidal behavior. It is beyond the scope of this book to discuss in detail the papers published on this subject as well as the methodological problems inherent in these studies. However, the methodological problems are to a certain extent identical to those in papers on suicidal behavior and somatic disorders.

Despite the above-mentioned reservation, it is necessary to give this review because many patients with somatic disorders also have mental disorders such as depression, anxiety disorders, or other psychological problems. Furthermore, suffering from a somatic disorder may also result in excessive use or abuse of tranquilizers, pain medication, or other stimulants. Suffering from a somatic disorder combined with a psychological problem often results in an increased risk of suicide. As an example, a review of all patients with multiple sclerosis who committed suicide in a certain period in Denmark showed that a large number of these patients also suffered from mental disorders or had problems due to drug or alcohol abuse (Stenager, Koch-Henriksen, and Stenager, 1996).

Different types of studies have been published that examine the relation between suicidal behavior and mental disorders. In the following, three types will be mentioned: studies based on forensic examinations, follow-up studies, and follow-up studies of patients with specific mental disorders.

1. *Studies based on forensic examinations.* People who committed suicide have been examined, and among those, the number of persons with psychiatric disorders has been determined based on interviews with relatives and doctors, as well as information on admittance to psychiatric wards.

   Such studies can have severe bias. It is not possible to use specific diagnostic criteria for a psychiatric disorder, and information from doctors, relatives, and hospital records may be insufficient. Deciding whether or not a causality exists is impossible because a previous mental disorder need not be associated with the actual suicide.

2. *Follow-up studies.* The frequency of mental disorders in patients who have attempted suicide has been estimated. After the attempt, the patients have been followed for a certain period of time, and the mental disorder as a risk factor in suicide has been determined. Such studies only give an estimation of the risk of suicide under the condition that a suicide attempt has been made and the person has a specific psychiatric disorder. The published studies have not always used comparable diagnostic criteria, and the populations may have been selected from a limited group, as an example, patients treated in psychiatric wards after a suicide attempt. Such a population never includes all suicide attempts. Furthermore, the follow-up periods are variable, and control groups and the statistics used may also result in bias.

3. *Follow-up studies of patients with specific mental disorders.* These are studies done on patients who have been admitted and/or treated for a mental disorder. The studies estimate the risk of suicide on the condition that the person has a specific disorder.

   This type of study also has methodological problems. Comparison of the studies can be difficult because variable diagnostic tools have been used, such as clinical diagnosis and rating scales research diagnostic criterias, i.e., DSM-III diagnosis. The treatments may differ widely. The follow-up periods vary and not all patients participate in the follow-up period. Furthermore, problems with control groups and statistics may occur.

In the next part of this chapter examples of the three types of studies are presented. More comprehensive information can be found in *Suicide*, edited by Alec Roy, which carefully presents descriptions of the influence of mental disorders on the risk of suicide.

FORENSIC STUDIES

In St. Louis during the period from 1956 to 1957, Robins and colleagues examined 134 suicides. Information about the suicides was consecutively collected and not selected. There was no control group. It was found that 94 percent of the persons had a mental disorder at the time of suicide. In twenty-five patients no diagnosis was made, 55 percent were depressed, and 28 percent abused alcohol. Anxiety or other neurotic disorders were not present in any of the patients.

In Seattle, Dorpat and Ripley (1960) examined 114 consecutive suicides in the period from 1957 to 1958. They found that 108 had a mental disorder. A little less than 30 percent suffered from depression, and 26.7 percent abused alcohol.

In the frequently quoted study by Barraclough and colleagues (1974) of 100 suicides in England during the period from 1966 to 1968, 93 percent had a mental disorder. Seventy percent were depressed, and 15 percent had abused alcohol. A further interesting point was that two-thirds had consulted their practitioner within a month before the suicide.

In Sweden, Beskow (1979) in the period 1970 to 1971 studied all male suicides, a total of 271. The suicides occurred in both urban and rural areas. The frequency of depression in urban areas was 45 percent and in rural areas 18 percent, while alcohol abuse occurred in 37 percent of the population in urban areas and only 18 percent in rural areas.

In Finland, Isometsa and colleagues (1993) from 1987 to 1988 selected a sample of 229 suicides from a total of 1,397. Diagnostic research criteria from the DSM-III-R were used, and it was determined 59 percent had depressive disorders while 43 percent abused alcohol.

Several other studies (Chynoweth, Tonnge, and Armstrong,

1980; Arato' et al., 1988; Maris, 1981; Rich, Young, and Fowler, 1986; Runeson, 1989; Åsgård, 1990) have confirmed the results in the previously quoted studies, i.e., a large percentage of persons committing suicide have suffered from a mental disorder, primarily depression and alcohol abuse.

Thus, the studies unanimously agree on the conclusion that many people who commit suicide have mental disorders, most frequently depression and alcohol abuse. The studies do not assess the risk of suicide when one suffers from a specific mental disorder, and in none of the studies have comparisons been made to mental disorders in relevant control groups.

RISK FACTORS OF SUICIDE IN PATIENTS WHO HAVE MADE A SUICIDE ATTEMPT

Numerous studies have been made in patients who have attempted suicide with the purpose of identifying risk factors for a later suicide. The studies have been described in reviews (Dorpat and Ripley, 1967; Lester, 1972; Brown and Sheran, 1972; van Egmond and Diekstra, 1990; Nielsen, 1994).

Typically, the studies have been performed in the following way. A cohort of suicide attempters have been selected and followed for five to ten years, and then the persons who eventually commit suicide have been identified. Thereafter, a comparison of the patients committing suicide and the suicide attempters have been made.

One of the recent large studies was made by Allgulander and Fisher in 1990. They followed 8,895 patients admitted due to self-poisoning in Stockholm during the period 1974 to 1985 in order to identify risk factors for suicide. In women, previous suicide attempts and personality disorders were predictors of suicide, while in men abuse of alcohol and drugs was an important risk factor. The study used modern and fine statistical methods.

Hawton and Fagg (1988) followed for eight years 1,959 persons who had attempted suicide. They also found that mental disorders (especially schizophrenia), abuse, bad health conditions, and previous suicide attempts were predictors of suicide.

Further Scandinavian studies of suicide attempters (Rygnestad,

1988; Suokas and Lønnquist, 1991; Nielsen, Wang, and Bille-Brahe, 1990) found that chronic neurotic disorders, alcohol and medication abuse, depression, and schizophrenia were suicide risk factors in suicide attempters. In a 1983 study of 1,018 suicide attempters who were treated in Helsinki after a suicide attempt, Soukas and Lønnquist found that 62 percent had been drinking alcohol prior to the attempt. After a five-and-one-half-year interim, the follow-up indicated that the yearly suicide rate was 598 per 100,000 in those who have been drinking alcohol. In the first year after the suicide attempt, the suicide rate was 1,809 per 100,000, equivalent of fifty-one times increased risk of suicide compared to the background population.

At the time of suicide, autopsy showed signs of chronic alcoholism in 30 percent of the patients who had been drinking in connection with a previous suicide attempt. Therefore, the authors recommended paying attention to alcohol consumption or abuse when treating suicide attempters.

The previous mentioned should have made it clear that almost all psychiatric disorders—depression, schizophrenia, personality disorders, chronic neurotic disorders, and abuse of alcohol and medication—result in an increased risk of suicide in those with prior attempts. Only few of the studies have used statistics that make it possible to evaluate the extent of the risk.

Many suicide attempters suffer from mental disorders. For example, Urwin and Gibbons (1979) used a standardized interview with 539 suicide attempters, and found that only 30 percent could be classified as not suffering from a mental disorder. Sixty percent were classified as depressed, but the depression was not as serious as in a comparable psychiatric-treated group of patients. Other studies (Ennis et al., 1989; Stenager, 1996) found that between one-fourth and one-third of suicide attempters could be classified as depressed.

Stenager used the DSM-III-R criteria to identify psychiatric disorders in persons admitted to a psychiatric ward after a suicide attempt and found that 31 percent were depressed, 10 percent suffered from other kinds of psychosis, 27 percent were alcohol abusers, 12 percent were drug abusers, 6 percent had anxiety disorders, and 37 percent had personality disorders. A total of 34 percent—41 percent of the women and 17 percent of the men—did not have a psychiatric disorder, which was in agreement with the study by Urwin and Gibbons (1979). The patients were selected and comprised the most severely disturbed suicide attempters. Therefore, the quoted figures must be considered maximum figures of mental disorders in suicide attempters.

FOLLOW-UP STUDIES
OF PSYCHIATRIC POPULATIONS

Numerous follow-up studies in psychiatric populations on the association of psychiatric disorders and suicide have been made. In 1977, Miles reviewed approximately 100 of such studies, among which thirty-four dealt with schizophrenia. In two studies (Bleuler, 1978; Tsuang, 1978), it was found that 12.9 percent and 10.1 percent of deaths among schizophrenics were due to suicide. Additionally, Miles concluded that approximately 10 percent of all schizophrenics commit suicide.

In 1985, Drake and colleagues reviewed the literature on suicide and schizophrenia, and specifically concentrated on areas that should be addressed in future studies. Despite the large number of studies, only few fulfilled accepted research criteria. Among the problems were lack of diagnostic criteria, lack of standardized methods of measurement, and limited focus—the studies just examined the hospital stay and not other life events. Prospective studies on cohorts of a defined group of patients followed for a number of years were recommended. Despite the methodological problems, Drake et al. concluded that young male schizophrenics were especially most vulnerable to self-destructive acts, particularly in the first years after onset of the disorder. Courses of the disorder that had frequent relapses increased the risk. Suicide occurred when the patient was depressed or felt that life was hopeless, but rarely in severely psychotic periods. The period after the patients were discharged from the hospital also had an accompanying increased risk of suicide.

Mortensen and Juel (1990) have studied mortality and causes of death in 6,178 Danish schizophrenic inpatients in the period 1957 to 1987. Generally, they found an increased risk of death in schizophrenic patients with a total Standard Mortality Ratio (SMR) of 1.23, and an increased risk of suicide with an SMR of 1.32. Due to the extensive and thorough Danish statistics on causes of death, the follow-up was almost complete. The study found just a slightly increased risk of suicide compared to other studies. This was explained by the fact that the study population was composed of chronic, long-term patients who survived the first years of the disorder, when the risk of suicide is highest. The surveillance of this group of patients was better than today because schizophrenic patients are now frequently treated as outpatients.

Monk (1987) has reviewed five large follow-up studies (Pokorny, 1983; Black, Warrack, and Winokur, 1985; Barner-Rasmussen, Dupont, and Bille, 1986; Babigian and Odoroff, 1969; Hagnell, Lanke, and Rorsman, 1981). The first three studies included admitted psychiatric patients, the fourth study included all patients receiving psychiatric treatment, and the fifth study included all inhabitants receiving psychiatric treatment in one town. The frequency of suicide varied from a ratio of 12.3 to 41.3. The patients with depressive disorders had the highest risk. One of the studies (Hagnell and Rorsmann, 1987) found that the risk of suicide in men with a mental disorder was thirty-nine times higher compared to men without a mental disorder. In men with depression, the number of suicides was eighty times higher compared to the number of suicides in men without a mental disorder.

Monk pointed out that the studies contained many methodological problems, including that the follow-up period varied, the quality of follow-up information varied, different sources of information (national registers, local registers, and others) were used, treatment possibilities ranged, and finally diagnostic criteria were diverse.

However, Monk concluded that there were strong reasons to believe that psychiatric disorders, and especially depression, were important risk factors for suicide. The risk was probably increased eight times or more.

Previously, we have dealt with studies mainly on depressive disorders, schizophrenia, and mental disorders in general. However, in the last few years, authors have studied and discussed whether or not anxiety/panic disorders and depressive neurotic disorders were associated with increased suicide risk.

In 1988, Coryell reviewed studies on panic disorders and suicide. He finally concluded that only a few studies dealt with this problem, and the risk of suicide in patients with panic disorders could be equivalent to the risk in depressed patients. The time span from when the diagnosis was made to the actual suicide might be longer in panic disorders. Coryell also acknowledged the possibility of comorbidity in the form of a secondary depression and abuse.

Based on a review of previous studies, Johnson, Weissman, and Klerman (1990) concluded that there was a similar risk of suicide in patients with panic disorders and depressive disorders. This was the case in both comorbidity and uncomplicated courses of both disorders. Friedman and colleagues (1992) tried to test this assertion by studying two populations with panic disorders and respectively with or without personality disorders and borderline personality disorder. They found that increased suicide risk was associated with a borderline personality, abuse, and affective instability. It was the consequences of the panic disorder more than the panic disorder per se that contributed to an increased suicide risk.

In 1994, Allgulander published a study that evaluated the association of panic disorder, depressive neurotic disorder, and mortality. The study included 9,912 patients with a panic disorder and 38,529 patients with a depressive neurotic disorder. The patients were identified in the National Psychiatric Case Register in Sweden in the time interval from 1973 to 1983. The Psychiatric Register was compared to the Swedish Register of causes of death. In men and women below forty-five years of age, the SMR of suicide in panic disorders was 6.7 and 4.9 respectively, and in depressive neurosis 12.6 and 15.7, respectively. The risk of suicide in both groups of disorders was significantly increased. The risk was highest during the first three months after discharge from the hospital. The study also demonstrated that the risk of suicide in patients with these disorders was higher than had been previously found in smaller studies. The study included many patients and used accepted statistical and methodological methods. Also, the Swedish population is homogenous and has equal access to treatment independent of social and economic conditions. These factors support the viability of the study's results. Finally, the study recommended an improved diagnostic method and treatment of patients with panic disorders.

CONCLUSION

Based on follow-up studies for ten to fifteen years in patients with depression, it has been estimated that approximately 15 percent commit suicide, leading to the conclusion that the lifetime risk of suicide in depressed patients is 15 percent (Guze and Robins, 1970). Studies on the association of alcohol and suicide are primarily based on forensic studies and populations of suicide attempters. The lifetime risk of suicide in alcoholics has been estimated at 10 to 15 percent, but studies designed to document this risk have been of poor quality and thus are inadequate (Murphy, 1986; Murphy and Wetzel, 1990).

The lifetime risk of suicide in schizophenics and patients with panic disorders is also increased by the presence of these disorders.

The lifetime risk of suicide in persons with depression, schizophrenia, and alcoholism is based on old studies. An accurate risk level has not been confirmed in recent studies with many patients using epidemiologically well-established research methods.

However, there is little doubt as pointed out by Monk, that having a mental disorder increases one's risk of suicide. The exact extent of the risk in a certain disorder is still unclear and will depend on the severity of the disorder, the options for treatment, the social network of the patient, and the comorbidity of other mental disorders. Finally, as the main theme in this book, suffering from a mental disorder and also having a somatic disorder associated with an increased risk of suicide further enhances the risk of suicide.

Frequently, professionals treating mental disorders pay little attention to their patients' somatic complaints. A lack of coordination of treatment can cause patients to feel frustrated and disappointed. Therefore, treatment professionals should be aware that not just mental disorders, but also somatic disorders, increase the risk of suicide. This is important when discussing prevention and treatment, and will be further discussed in the last chapter.

Chapter 4

Methodological Problems

As already described, the risk of suicide is increased in patients with mental disorders, such as schizophrenia and manic-depressive psychosis (Mortensen and Juel, 1990).

In patients with various somatic disorders, the risk of having a mental disorder is substantially increased, compared to healthy persons. For example, patients with certain neurological disorders, such as multiple sclerosis, epilepsy, cerebral stroke, and Parkinson's disease, have an increased risk of depression.

Patients with other somatic disorders, such as heart disease, and endocrinological disorders, such as diabetes mellitus, also have an increased risk of mental disorders, especially depression.

Barraclough (1987) and Guze and Robins (1970) have estimated the lifetime risk of committing suicide as approximately 15 percent in patients with depressions. Comparing this with the increased risk of depression in patients with somatic disorders, it is to be expected that patients with a somatic disorder also have an increased risk of suicide compared to the general population.

Patients who have disorders involving pain also have an increased risk of having a mental disorder. Consequently, patients who experience chronic pain are also expected to have an increased risk of suicide (Fishbain et al., 1991).

Obviously, if suicide is to be prevented in patients with somatic disorders, it is important to know which groups of patients and which disorders are associated with an increased risk of suicide. Furthermore, it is important to know when in the course of the disorder and in which age groups the risk of suicide is greatest. The literature dealing with the risk of suicidal behavior in patients with somatic disorders is comprehensive (Whitlock, 1982; Stensman and

Sundqvist-Stensman, 1988). Previous reviews on somatic disorders and risk of suicide have rarely been critical toward the methods used in the design of the studies.

However, the studies use various methods, which make comparisons difficult, and perhaps impossible, and the results should not be considered conclusive. Consequently, before a presentation is made of results from previous studies on the risk of suicidal behavior in patients with somatic disorders and pain—as will be made in the next chapters—a careful review of the methodological problems in these studies is necessary.

METHODOLOGICAL PROBLEMS IN EVALUATING SUICIDAL RISK

When the risk of suicidal behavior is evaluated in patients with somatic disorders, a number of problems arise, including the following (Stenager and Stenager, 1992):

- Which type of study has been chosen?
- How is the study population defined and selected?
- Which control groups have been used in comparative studies?
- Which epidemiological and statistical methods have been used?
- Is an over- or underregistration of suicides possible? Can we trust the suicide statistics?

Choice of Type of Study

Usually, one of the following three types of studies has been used:

1. *Autopsy studies.* These studies are primarily based on forensic information on deceased patients. Typically, the number of patients with a specific disorder who have committed suicide has been counted.
2. *Follow-up studies.* These studies count the number of patients committing suicide among those who have been admitted due to a specific disorder in a specific ward at a hospital in a defined period of time.

3. *Register studies.* These studies are based on a register of a defined population of patients. In such studies, it is possible to compare the diagnosed patients in the register to the cause of death statistics in a particular region (county, state, country) in a defined period of time. Then it is possible to calculate the number of suicides among the patients and in the background population. Comparing the two ratios, it is possible to calculate the relative risk. A relative risk of 1.5 means a 50 percent increased risk of death compared to the background population.

If a standardization of age is made, then it is possible to calculate the standardized mortality ratio (SMR), which is a measure of the relative risk. An SMR of 2 means a doubled risk of death.

Studies based on *autopsy materials*, i.e., forensic studies, present a special problem: it is very difficult to find a representative control group. Most autopsy studies comprise selected populations of patients, i.e., patients examined by forensic doctors and patients admitted to hospitals. Some studies have tried to overcome this problem by comparing the frequency of the disorder in the study and in the population. As a result, deceased and living persons are compared. Furthermore, the distribution of age and gender in the two populations is not expected to be the same. Consequently, conclusions drawn from such studies must be taken with reservation.

The most accurate study populations are major registers, which cover a large group of patients with a specific illness, including patients in various stages of the illness. Only by using such a population is it possible to estimate the risk of suicide for all patients with the disorder. By using large registers, an optimal statistical and epidemiological method can be used in evaluating the risk of suicide. The problem is, however, that only a few of these registers exist. Thus, optimal studies are often impossible to conduct for most disorders.

Only a few countries, for example the Scandinavian countries, have such registers including all persons in the country with the disorder. Consequently, register-based studies on suicidal behavior are difficult to perform.

All Scandinavian countries have registers on cancer, but in some of the countries, registers on neurological disorders (such as multiple sclerosis) and mental disorders also exist. Furthermore, it is possible to make registers on defined populations of patients. Finally, in a number of countries, whole population registers exist; thus, information concerning all patients with defined disorders can be obtained.

In the Scandinavian countries, the populations are homogeneous, registers exist, and health care is publicly funded. Therefore, it is possible to perform studies on well-defined, homogeneous, and complete populations.

As will be presented in the following chapters, many of the methodologically fine studies with many patients have been made by Scandinavian researchers (Allgulander and Fisher, 1990; Stenager, Brille-Brahe, and Jensen, 1991; Stenager et al., 1992).

Study Population

Definition of the Disorder

Before studying the association between a certain disorder and the risk of suicide, it is important that the disorder is well defined, and that strict and exact definitions of the diagnosis exist.

In a number of studies, the disorders have not been defined exactly or criteria for the presence of the disorder were not made. This has especially been a problem in studies on epilepsy, where the risk of suicide is increased in patients with certain types of seizures (Barraclough, 1987).

Small Populations

Many studies encompass only small populations, frequently approximately 100 patients. Suicide is a rare occurrence, e.g., in the United States, where the suicide rate is 10 to 13 per 100,000 persons; however, in Denmark the rate is 30 per 100,000, which is one of the highest suicide rates next to Finland and Japan. Therefore, if only small populations are studied, the results are inaccurate.

Selection

A major problem in many studies is selection. Frequently, the study population consists of patients admitted to a special-care unit. Thus, such study-populations comprise the most ill patients, and generalizing the results to all patients with the disorder would be inaccurate.

Another selection problem is the patients excluded, for example, due to uncertainty of the cause of death. If this is not handled properly, the statistics will be biased.

Control Groups

Frequently, the general population is used as a control group, when researchers are evaluating suicide risk. However, in a number of studies, it has not been taken into account that the risk of suicide varies with both age and gender. Older people have a higher risk of suicide than young people, and men a higher risk than women. On the other hand, young persons have a higher risk of parasuicide (suicide attempt) than older persons, and women have a higher risk of parasuicide than men. Depending on the age and gender distribution of the studied population, it is possible both to over- and underestimate the risk of suicide. Furthermore, if a small population is used, a major risk of bias exist.

The problem of control groups also exist, when comparing them with autopsy studies, as previously mentioned.

Methods of Statistics

Different statistical methods have been used in the suicide studies quoted in the following chapters.

1. Based on the risk of suicide in the background-population, a calculation of the observed and expected number of deaths is made.
2. A comparison of the percentage of patients committing suicide with a specific disorder to a control group is made.
3. Based on the risk of suicide in the background and studied population, an age-, and gender-standardized mortality ratio (SMR) is calculated. This is considered the best statistical method.

Due to the different methods used, comparison of various studies is very difficult. In reviews, comparisons of selected materials have been made, and wrong conclusions have been the result.

Finally, a number of case stories exist, but obviously no general conclusions can be based on such cases.

Validity of Suicide Statistics

In patients with a severe somatic disorder, it is to be expected that death will perhaps not be registered as suicide or a possible suicide, but as a natural death. This risk exists especially in communities where suicide is considered taboo for religious or other reasons. Thus, the risk of suicide can be underestimated, making the statistics in a number of countries are hardly valid, especially concerning a controversial cause of death such as suicide.

In other countries, well-organized registers and health care exist, and consequently valid and complete registers of causes of death should be expected. But even in such countries, problems of validity have been documented. When evaluating results of studies on suicide risk these problems of validity should be considered.

A concluding remark would be that studies on the risk of suicide in patients with chronic disorders should be evaluated carefully, regarding the methods used, before decisive conclusions on the presence of increased risk of suicide are made.

Chapter 5

Suicide in Patients
with Neurological Disorders

GENERAL RISK OF SUICIDE
IN NEUROLOGICAL DISORDERS

In several studies, attempts have been made to estimate the risk of suicide in patients with various diseases, including neurological disorders, in large populations by reviewing forensic studies.

Whitlock (1985) reviewed 1,000 suicides in England and Wales in the period from 1968 to 1972. He compared the number of suicides in persons with a certain disorder with the frequency of the disorder in the background population. He found a significantly increased risk of suicide in persons with epilepsy, multiple sclerosis, brain injuries, and brain tumors.

Stensman and Sundqvist-Stensman (1988) examined 416 suicides in Sweden in the period from 1977 to 1984 using the same methodological approach. They also found an increased risk of suicide in persons with neurological disorders.

The methods used in the two studies, i.e., comparing the frequency of illness in persons committing suicide with the frequency of the illness in the background population, can hardly justify the conclusions made in the studies. Among other, it is probably not possible to assume that the age- and sex-distribution in the general population is the same as in the population committing suicide. Besides that, varying mortality rates for persons suffering from the disorders studied, will also influence the results.

Allgulander and Fisher (1990) made a follow-up study in a representative sample of all patients admitted after self-poisoning in Stockholm in the period from 1974 to 1985. An attempt was made to identify predictors for future suicidal behavior, i.e., both suicide attempts and suicides. One of the findings was that a neurological disorder increased the risk of repeated suicide attempts. However, only few men with a neurological disorder were included in the study. So the result could be a casual finding, which should be examined closer in order to be confirmed.

The mentioned studies indicate an increased suicide risk associated with neurological disorders. In the following, the suicide risk in persons with various neurological disorders will be reviewed.

MULTIPLE SCLEROSIS

Multiple sclerosis (MS) is a disorder of the white matter of the brain. Despite the fact that the disorder has been known for more than 150 years, the cause is still unknown. It is believed that external factors can trigger the disorder in predisposed persons, causing breakdown (demyelination) of nerve fibers due to changes in the immunological system in the brain. Usually, the patients initially have attacks of the disease, i.e., symptoms may be present for days, weeks, or months and then disappear. Later on, the disease may have a progressive course, i.e., the impairment increases but the attacks disappear. For some patients, the end result may be severe disability.

The symptoms are varied, but may include visual disturbances, coordination problems, paresis, sensory disturbances, urinary problems, mental changes, memory problems, and sexual changes and problems. The onset most frequently occurs at a young age, i.e., in one's twenties or thirties. Women are more frequently affected than men, and, to date, no cure exists. However, in the last few years, treatments have been introduced that temporarily may slow down the progression of the disorder. (See Chapter 2 for a more thorough discussion of MS.)

Whether or not multiple sclerosis is associated with an increased risk of suicide has been examined in a number of studies (Table 5.1).

In the studies by Müller (1949); McAlpine, Lumsden, and Acheson (1972); Schwartz and Pierron (1972), and Kurtzke (1970) no increased risk of suicide was found. Their results were based on a small number of patients.

TABLE 5.1. Suicide Risk in Patients with Multiple Sclerosis

Author	Period	Number	Number of Suicides	Autopsy Study	Follow-Up Study	SMR	Increased Risk	Comments
Schwartz and Pierron	1972	408	4	yes	no	no	no	No adequate statistical method used
Sadovnick et al.	1972-1988	3,126	18	yes	no	no	yes	Control group not sex-adjusted
Kurtzke	1942-1951	476	1	no	yes	no	no	No calculation of suicide risk
Stenager et al. (1992)	1953-1985	6,088	58	no	yes	1.83	yes	Correct statistical method
Leibowitz, Kahana, and Alter	1960-1966	295	8	no	yes	no	yes	

Leibowitz, Kahana, and Alter (1971) found in a study conducted in Israel that the risk of suicide was increased fourteen times in patients with multiple sclerosis. In a Canadian study, Sadovnick and colleagues (1985) found thirteen suicides among eighty deceased MS patients. A Danish pilot study (Stenager, Stenager, and Jensen, 1991) comprised of MS patients admitted to a university hospital in the period from 1973 to 1985 found that 5 of 56 deaths were due to suicide. In none of the quoted studies was an age- or sex-standardized comparison with the general population made.

The largest, and from a methodological point of view most correctly, conducted study concerning the risk of suicide in MS patients is from Denmark (Stenager et al., 1992). The study is based on approximately 5000 patients registered in the Danish MS Registry. Standardized mortality ratios were calculated. Results showed that men diagnosed with MS before the age of forty years had a 3.12 increased risk of committing suicide, and women diagnosed before the age of forty years had a 2.12 increased risk of suicide compared to the general population. Patients diagnosed after the age of forty years did not have an increased risk of suicide. The risk of suicide was significantly increased within the first five years after the diagnosis was made. The total lifetime risk of committing suicide was approximately twice that of the general population.

In a Canadian study, Sadovnick and colleagues (1985) found a significantly higher risk of suicide, i.e., a 7.5 increased risk of suicide. However, the standardized mortality ratio had not been calculated, nor had a sex standardization been made, resulting in a considerable bias due to the skewed sex distribution in patients with MS.

The final conclusion, based on the most recent studies, is that patients with MS have an increased risk of suicide, but the risk is moderate and confined to younger patients.

EPILEPSY

Epilepsy is actually the symptom of a temporary electrical dysfunction (depolarization) of the nerve fibers in the brain. The presentation of the symptoms is dependent on which part of the brain is involved. The depolarization, which generates the seizures, may start in some of the deep structures of the brain or in the cortical areas. As a result, the seizures may either involve loss of consciousness and perhaps be accompanied by spasms in arms and legs or preserved consciousness and only convulsions. Seizures generated from the temporal lobes may be associated with changed behavior and eventually mental disturbances such as psychosis.

Epilepsy is one of the most frequent neurological disorders. The cause of epilepsy is complex. In a simplified description, the cause can be either due to changes in the transmitters in the nervous system or due to structural changes.

Nerve transmitters transfer impulses from one nerve fiber to another. Changes in this system may be due to failures during the development of the brain or genetically inherited changes, but frequently the cause is unknown.

Structural changes may be scars after brain injuries, brain infections, brain hemorrhages, stroke damage, or tumors.

Epilepsy is found in both children and adults. It can afflict otherwise healthy persons, or it can be associated with other mental disabilities. Consequently, the prognosis and social implications are very diverse. These aspects have to be acknowledged when we are discussing suicide risk in epilepsy.

Finally, a large number of treatments exist and they are continuously being improved, but in spite of that, about one-fourth of epilepsy patients may not be seizure-free.

Concerning the association between illness and suicide, epilepsy is one of the most carefully examined disorders (Table 5.2).

In 1941 Prudhomme published a study comprised of 75,000 admittances of patients with epilepsy, and he found 67 suicides. Due to the methods used, the study only confirmed that suicides did occur in patients with this disorder, but the frequency could not be estimated.

A Danish study from 1970 by Henriksen, Juul-Jensen, and Lund examined the mortality among a representative large group of patients with epilepsy. They found that the risk of suicide was increased three times.

In Poland, Zielinski (1974) examined Warsaw residents with epilepsy. In the period from 1967 to 1969, 239 deaths occurred. The risk of suicide was increased five times in men and ten times in women. In a Finnish study by Ivanainen and Lehtimen of 179

TABLE 5.2. Suicide Risk in Epileptic Patients

Author	Period in years	Number	Number of suicides	Comments
Prudhomme	undefined	75,000	67	No increased risk. The study confirmed the presence of suicide in this particular group.
Henriksen, Juul-Jensen, and Lund	1950-1964	2,763	21	Risk increased three times. The control group selected from low-risk persons. No age or sex adjustment.
Zielenski	1965-1969	6,710	12	Risk increased. Males 5 times, females ten times. Undefined control group. No age or sex adjustment.
White, McLean, and Howland	1931-1971	2,000	21	Mortality ratio = 5.4. Age-adjusted study.
Ivanainen and Lehtimen	1900-1976	179	13	Risk increased three times. Strongly selected high risk population. No age or sex adjustment.

deaths of previously admitted epileptics, thirteen were found to be due to suicide, which was significantly more than in the general population. The study group was highly selected.

None of these studies contained information on age and sex standardization. Therefore, the conclusions were uncertain.

In a follow-up study, White, McLean, and Howland (1979) examined 2,000 patients admitted to the Center of Epilepsy at Chalfont between 1931 and 1971, and treated with anticonvulsant therapy. The study ended in 1977. The risk of suicide was compared to the general population. An age- and sex-standardization was made, and the time at risk has been taken into consideration. White, McLean, and Howland (1979) found that the risk of suicide was increased 5.4 times. From a methodological point of view, this is one of the most accurately conducted studies.

In 1981 Matthews and Barabas reviewed the literature on the association between suicide risk and epilepsy. They reviewed a large number of small studies on deaths in selected groups of epilepsy patients in different countries. The accumulated risk of suicide in these studies was 5 percent. This was compared to the risk of suicide in the American population of 1.4 percent. The result was interpreted as an indication of an increased risk of suicide in epilepsy patients.

Barraclough (1987) made a comprehensive review of the existing literature suicide risk in epileptic patients who have different kinds of seizures. He found that patients who had seizures that generated from the temporal lobes were 5 times more at risk for suicide. Patients with treatment refractory seizures, i.e., patients who were not seizure-free, were twenty-five times more risk for suicide.

The methods used in the last two reviews are subjected to criticism. They cannot be used as definitive documentation of an increased risk of suicide in epileptics because accumulated number of deaths from a large number of selected patients in different countries have been used.

The final conclusion is that one of the quoted studies is methodologically correct—the one by White, McLean, and Howland, 1979—but the remaining studies have a substantial number of possibilities for making wrong conclusions regarding the extent of the increased risk of suicide in epileptics in general as well as in groups of patients with different kinds of seizures.

White, McLean, and Howland found a 5.4 times increased risk of suicide in treated patients. Since then, no studies have been conducted, but improved treatment possibilities (pharmacologically, surgical, and socially) may be expected to have reduced the risk of suicide in this disorder.

HUNTINGTON'S CHOREA

Huntington's chorea is an autosomal dominant inherited disorder, which means that if a person is afflicted by the disorder, the risk that the offspring also becomes ill is 50 percent. The gene responsible for the disorder is located on the short arm of chromosome 4.

Huntington's chorea is a disorder characterized by a progressive degeneration of specific parts of the brain. The onset usually occurs during a person's thirties and forties, and on the average, the afflicted individual will live 10 to 20 years with the disorder.

The symptoms are a gradually changed personality, mental symptoms such as dementia, and physical symptoms such as involuntary movements and dyscoordination. Currently, a cure does not exist.

The first description was made by Huntington in 1872. He clearly stated that mental symptoms were part of the disorder and that a considerable risk existed that afflicted individuals would commit suicide.

Regarding the risk of suicide, this disorder presents a unique problem. Due to the autosomal inheritance, patients know the consequences of the disorder from close family members. They know that they have a 50 percent risk of getting the disorder, and they consider this when choosing their education, planning future opportunities, and deciding whether or not to have children.

Using genetic tests, it is now possible to identify persons who will become ill later in life. The result of this has very severe ethical, moral, and human considerations concerning how to adapt to this possibility. Obviously, some persons will be relieved by learning that they do have the disorder, but others will have to face the fact that they will eventually become ill.

Interview studies of persons at risk have been performed. In one of those studies (Kessler, 1987), sixty-seven persons with either a mother or father with Huntington's chorea were interviewed. Forty percent of the interviewed persons had experienced suicidal behavior in the family, and 78.8 percent wanted to know whether or not they had the disorder, if it was possible. Seventy-one percent would undergo an abortion if their fetus was a carrier of the Huntington's chorea gene. Finally, 11 percent mentioned suicide as a possibility if their test results indicated Huntington's chorea.

Such a test must have a high predictive value, i.e., a low risk of obtaining false positive and false negative test results. Furthermore, the consequence of a screening of risk groups could be an increased risk of suicide.

Studies on the risk of suicide in patients with Huntington's chorea and their relatives are reviewed in Table 5.3.

TABLE 5.3. Suicide Risk in Patients with Huntington's Chorea

Author	Period	Number of Participants	Number of Suicides	Autopsy Study	Follow-Up Study	Increased Risk	Comments
Reed and Chandler	1940-1956	203	3	No	Yes		Small population. No age or sex adjustment.
Schoenfeld et al.	1980-1983	506	20	Yes		under 50 years OR = 1.06 over 50 years OR = 8.19	Selection due to unsure cause of death for one-third of the population.
Saugstad and Ødegård	1916-1975	199	1	No	Yes	No	Selected psychiatric population. Use high-risk population as controls.
Farrer	undefined	452	5.7% of all deaths	Yes		Increased 4 times	No age adjustment. A large number of dropouts.

*OR = Odds Ratio

39

From a number of sources, Reed and Chandler (1958) gathered patients who had been diagnosed as suffering from Huntington's chorea. The patients were followed from 1940 to 1956. Two studies were made: a study of suicides in families with Huntington's chorea and a study of patients living with the disease in 1940.

In the first study of family members, an increased risk of suicide was found compared to the normal population, i.e., three times for men and five times for women. The results of a second study on patients with Huntington's chorea did not indicate an increased risk of suicide (Reed and Chandler, 1958). In the quoted studies, problems existed in the selection of the population. The population was small, and age standardization was not made. Consequently, the increased mortality must be interpretated with caution.

Shoenfeld and colleagues studied 506 patients, among which 403 had a definite diagnosis and 103 a possible diagnosis. They found twenty suicides in the population, corresponding to a five times increased risk of suicide in patients above fifty years of age, but no increased risk in patients below fifty years. However, the cause of death was only established with certainty in one-third of the studied patients, which means that the the risk of suicide may have been underestimated. As a consequence, the authors also have examined those patients whose cause of death was established with certainty. In this group, the risk of suicide was increased three times in persons below fifty years of age, and twenty-three times in persons above fifty years.

In Norway, Saugstad, and Ødegård examined all patients with Huntington's chorea admitted to psychiatric departments from 1916 to 1975. One suicide and one suicide attempt was found in this study. Calculated from the yearly number of suicides in psychiatric departments, the expected number of suicides would be two. The conclusion from the study should be that patients with Huntington's chorea do not have a higher risk of suicide than other patients admitted to psychiatric departments, and *not* as the authors claim, that suicide is rare. Due to a methodological error, they use a high-risk group as the control group.

Farrer (1986) examined 452 patients with Huntington's chorea, and found that 5.7 percent of the deaths were due to suicide. This result was compared to the risk of suicide in the Canadian and

American population of 1.5 percent, corresponding to a four times increased risk in patients with Huntington's chorea. Those persons who committed suicide had at least survived half of their expected survival time after onset the disease.

Thus, most studies document an increased risk of suicide in patients with Huntington's chorea, but all studies have bias, which means that the validity of the test results must be taken with reservation.

SPINAL CORD AND BRAIN INJURIES

Spinal Cord Injuries

Spinal cord injuries are frequently caused by accidents such as diving in shallow water, motorcycle accidents, or car crashes. In these accidents, the spinal cord is crushed or torn. The symptoms depend on which level the spinal cord is injured. The symptoms include paralysis, numbness, loss of control of bladder and bowel functions, change or loss of sexual function, and eventually infertility. If the injury encompass the cervical spine, artificial respiration may be necessary.

The victims are most often young men. Those afflicted have to face life in a wheelchair, perhaps connected to a respirator. They are primarily dependent on the help of other people and have reduced possibilities of education and raising families.

Nyquist and Bors (1967) studied 2,011 patients admitted to an American hospital in the period 1946 to 1965. (See Table 5.4.) Twenty-one patients committed suicide, equivalent of 1.3 percent of all patients and 8.1 percent of all deaths. The majority of the suicides was in young patients less than thirty years old.

Geisler and colleagues (1983) and Geisler, Jousse, and Wynne-Jones (1983) have made two studies on mortality in patients with spinal cord injuries. The first study covered the period from 1945 to 1973 and included 1,501 patients, while the second study covered the period from 1973 to 1980. The studies described a representative group of patients who had survived an accident. An increased risk of suicide compared to the general population was found. The

TABLE 5.4. Suicide Risk in Patients with Spinal Lesions

Author	Period in Years	Number of Participants	Number of Suicides	Follow-Up Study	Increased Risk	SMR	Comments
Nyquist and Bors	1946-1965	2,011	21	Yes	Yes	No	The highest number of suicides among the young < 30 years. No risk assessment.
Geisler, Jousse, and Wynne-Jones	1945-1973	1,501	18	Yes	Yes	No	Suicide risk increased. Decrease in mortality.
Geisler et al.	1973-1980	1,510	21	Yes	Yes	No	Age-adjusted normal population.
Le and Price	1963-1976	417	6	Yes	Yes	No	Suicide the second most common cause of death. Most frequent among quadriplegic patients.
Frisbie and Kache	1973-1982	923	5	Yes	Yes, among the young, four times.	No	Use age- but not sex-adjusted normal population. Newly diagnosed patients.
DeVivo et al.	1973-1984	9,135	50	Yes	Yes	4.9	Correct statistical method.

risk of suicide increased along with the falling general mortality in the period after the injury.

A study by Le and Price (1982) examined 417 patients with a spinal cord lesion in the period from 1963 to 1976. A careful calculation of the survival of the patients compared to an age- and gender-matched population was made. As expected, an increased mortality was found among patients with spinal cord injuries. However, along with an increasing survival time due to better treatment options, a remarkable finding was that suicide was the second most frequent cause of death in this group, and suicide was the most frequent cause of death in patients with quadriplegia, i.e., paralysis of both legs and arms.

In the period from 1973 to 1982, Frisbie and Kache (1983) followed 923 patients, among whom 132 died. A comparison with an age-standardized control group disclosed an increased mortality among young, but not older patients. The risk of suicide was estimated to be four times of the general population, and was highest among younger and newly diagnosed patients.

In order to identify patients with spinal cord lesions at risk of committing suicide, Charlifue and Gerhart (1991) have compared forty-two patients with spinal cord injuries who committed suicide with a control group whose members did not commit suicide and matched for age, gender, and level of spinal cord lesion. The identified risk factors did not differ from risk factors found in other patient groups who had committed suicide, i.e., patients who previously had attempted suicide. DeVivo and colleagues (1991) studied 9,135 injured persons between 1973 and 1984. The SMR was 4.9. The highest SMR occurred one to five years after the injury.

In conclusion, patients with spinal cord injuries have higher mortality rates than the general population. Suicide is one of the most frequent causes of death in this population, and it is assumed that the risk of suicide is increased four times compared to the background population. The highest risk is found among young patients, patients with quadriplegia, and newly diagnosed patients. From a methodological point of view, the quality of the studies is acceptable.

Brain Injuries

Brain damage can occur from many reasons. Brain injures can be caused by trauma to the head, which may occur in traffic accidents, falls, fightings, and wars. Brain injuries occur in people of all ages and in both genders, but most frequently in young and middle-aged men. The symptoms and permanent impairment depend on the extent and location of the damage. This means that some patients do not have permanent impairment while others have paresis and/or spasticity in combination with personality changes and cognitive deficits such as memory impairment. Symptomatic epilepsy may also result. In some patients, mental and cognitive changes may be the dominant symptoms. Consequently, patients with brain injuries are a very heterogeneous group.

Only few studies exist on the risk of suicide in patients with brain injuries, and most of these studies were conducted in the 1960s.

In a comprehensive Finnish study, Achté, Lönnquist, and Hillbom (1971) studied 6,498 Finnish men suffering from brain injury during the the Finnish War from 1939 to 1945. They found 107 (9.1 percent) of the deceased to have committed suicide. In the first twenty-five years after the injury, the suicide rate was 70 to 80/100,000 per year. This was twice the suicide rate in the normal population. The suicide rate in patients with brain injuries who afterward had suffered from a psychosis was 400/100,000. Patients with severe injuries, open injuries, and symptomatic epilepsy as a complication had an extensively higher suicide risk. The suicide risk was low in the first year after the injury, and then increased.

Vaukonen (1959) also made a follow-up study on soldiers from the Finnish War (1939-1945). Among 3,700 soldiers with brain injuries, thirty-seven committed suicide prior to 1957, equaling 14 percent of all deaths. The purpose of the study was not to estimate suicide risk, but to clarify the soldiers' conditions, which could explain the suicide. Frequently, the impairment was so severe that the patient had to give up his previous occupation. Some patients experienced increasing impairment, and some had psychological problems before suffering from the injury. Other patients had psychotic episodes after the injury, and two patients committed suicide while they were psychotic.

In a third study, Lewin, Marshall, and Roberts (1979) made a twenty-five-year follow-up study on 479 patients with brain injuries who were comatose or had amnesia for a week or more after the injury. In this study, three committed suicide, but the expected number was one.

All the studies on brain injuries are on victims from World War II; no up-to-date studies have been made on suicide in patients with brain injuries. Better options for treatment and psychosocial support for patients with brain injuries would most likely decrease the suicide risk.

BRAIN TUMORS

Brain tumors occur in both children and adults. In adults the tumors have onset in the third decade and afterward. Metastatic tumors, i.e., tumors spread from others organs, usually present in the sixth or seventh decade. The location of the tumors decides the presentation of symptoms, but most frequently the first symptom is an epileptic seizure.

Meningeomas are benign tumors that usually can be surgically removed and perhaps supplemented with radiation therapy. Other tumors are benign, but may transform to malignant tumors, and finally, malignant tumors are associated with such a bleak prognosis. The prognosis for metastatic tumors depends on the parent tumor.

Brain tumors can be associated with epilepsy, mental changes, and cognitive deficits as well a number of other symptoms, and thus will have profound influence on daily living.

In a review of the literature in 1932, Henry found that approximately 10 percent of patients with brain tumors had suicidal impulses. In a 1938 study by Keschner, Bender, and Strauss of 530 patients, just a few with suicidal behavior were found.

In a case story, the suicide of a patient with a nondiagnosed meningeoma was described (Feigin, 1988). However, a number of studies on the association of cancer and suicide have been performed (Stenager, Jensen, and Bille-Brahe, 1991), and an increased risk of suicide in cancer patients has been found. However, in none of these studies has an increased suicide risk been documented in patients with brain tumors compared to other cancer patients.

Furthermore, a major problem exists when studying suicide risk in patients with tumors because the length of survival for malignant tumors is short and impairment is rapid. Therefore, the risk of suicide is expected to be low—and difficult to measure. On the other hand, survival time for patients with benign tumors is expected to be long. In spite of this fact, no studies have been performed.

PARKINSON'S DISEASE

Parkinson's disease, also named "shaking palsy," was first described in 1817 by James Parkinson. The disorder is a common neurological disorder, usually with onset in the fifties or later, and is found in both men and women. The symptoms are tremors, rigidity, and bradykinesia, i.e., slow movements. The symptoms are due to changes in the transmitter system in structures (basal ganglia) in the deep part of the brain. The symptoms can be alleviated medically, at least for a number of years. Experiments on transplanting fetal grafts as a potential treatment are ongoing, and tremors can be alleviated surgically in some patients. The expected life span due to the disease is only shortened a few years.

In Parkinson's disease, mental changes may also occur; thus some patients become demented. Depression occurs, and it has been estimated that 30 to 50 percent of patients with Parkinson's disease will suffer from depression (Mayeux et al., 1984). Furthermore, a transmitter—the serotonin metabolite 5-HIAA—that is associated with depression has been found to be decreased in patients with Parkinson's disease. Consequently, it could be hypothisized that the disorder could be associated with an increased suicide risk.

Only one study on the risk of suicide in patients with Parkinson's disease has been performed (Stenager et al., 1994). In this study, 485 patients who were treated in a neurological department participated. The risk of suicide in Parkinson's disease in men was significantly lower and in women at the same level as in the background population. High age at onset and good treatment possibilities were thought to be the explanation of the low suicide risk.

A few case stories also exist. In 1967 Hoehn and Yahr published a study on the mortality of 802 patients treated from 1949 to 1964 in a department with special interest in Parkinson's disease. Among the 340 deceased, three had committed suicide. No comparison with the risk of suicide in the background population was made.

In a similar study by Schneider and colleagues (1981), three among 127 deaths were due to suicide.

Finally, Jackson, Free, and Pike (1923) and Mindham (1970) have described the psychiatric disorders associated with Parkinson's disease, but concluded that they were superseded by the neurological symptoms. Obviously, they should be acknowledged and treated properly.

CEREBRAL STROKE

Cerebral stroke includes both hemorrhage and thrombosis or infarction. A hemorrhage is an excessive discharge of blood from a blood vessel. This can be either an arterial or venous bleeding. Both types can be fatal, but subarachnoidal hemorrhage is especially feared.

A thrombosis is usually in the arterial system, but can also occur in the venous system. The thrombosis can be due to a local clotting of the cells in the blood or due to an embolism from another part of the vascular system, such as the heart or carotid artery.

The symptoms depend on which part of the brain is affected. Patients may recover completely or have minor or major deficits. Thrombosis usually occurs in older people while subarachnoidal bleeding can occur in young or middle-aged people.

Despite stroke being the most frequent neurological disorder, only few inadequate studies on suicide risk in stroke patients exist. Oyebode, Kennedy, and Davidson (1986) studied twenty patients with subarachnoidal hemorrhage and psychiatric disorder. Two patients committed suicide and three made serious suicide attempts. The patients were selected. Consequently, the risk of suicide could not be estimated.

Garden, Garrison, and Jain (1990) and Folstein, Maiberger, and McHugh (1977) have found a considerably increased risk of depressive disorders in patients with cerebral strokes. Therefore, they recommend a careful clinical evaluation regarding depressive disorder, and caution awareness of the risk of suicide.

Finally, a study is currently being conducted by Stenager, Madsen, Stenager, and Boldsen, which will document a significantly increased suicide risk among stroke patients.

AMYOTROPHIC LATERAL SCLEROSIS (MOTOR NEURON DISEASE)

Amyotrophic lateral sclerosis or motor neuron disease is a rare progressive degenerative disease of the motor neuron system. The transmission of impulses from the spinal cord to the peripheral nervous system is gradually blocked, resulting in muscle weakness, muscle wasting, muscle fasciculation, speech problems, swallowing problems, and finally wasting of the respiratory muscles. The cause of the disease is unknown. Recent studies have documented that 15 percent of the diseased have an inherited form. The onset is usually in mid life. The disease is usually fatal within three years. No cure exists.

Only one study has been performed on the risk of suicide in motor neuron disease. In this study 116 patients participated. No association between suicide and the disorder was found.

CONCLUSION

The presented critical review of the literature on suicidal behavior in patients with neurological disorders has shown that the conclusions in previous studies were not based on solid facts due to the small number of patients studied and methodological problems. This is especially obvious in the studies on epilepsy, Huntington's chorea, and brain injuries.

In epilepsy, a number of seizure types or syndromes exist. One way of estimating the risk of suicide would be to consider the risk in each syndrome per se. As an example, syndromes associated with mental symptoms such as psychosis would be expected to have a higher risk. The alternative would be to study representatively selected groups of patients. A major obstacle to such studies is that epilepsy patients usually are treated in many different settings.

Huntington's chorea illustrates another obstacle that may hinder conclusive studies. Studies should include the period during which people are at risk to incur the disorder, i.e., the prediagnostic period. One of the Huntington's chorea studies showed that the risk of suicide was higher in this period than after the disease was diagnosed.

The studies on spinal cord injuries and multiple sclerosis are of sufficient quality to justify the conclusion that these disorders are associated with an increased risk of suicide. Regarding spinal cord injuries, mortality studies with survival analysis on large groups of patients have been made. However, estimation of the extent of suicide risk has not been performed. In multiple sclerosis, an increased suicide risk has been documented in a nationwide study covering the population of all MS patients, i.e., a optimally performed methodological study.

The studies on brain injuries are on victims from World War II; thus, we have no recent studies and no studies on patients with brain injuries caused by traffic accidents. It could be argued that getting hurt in a war where there were insufficient medical facilities is an extreme situation that would enhance the risk of suicide. Thus, studies on the risk in victims of traffic accidents who hopefully have better options of sufficient treatment would be most welcome. Furthermore, the previous studies were not matched with a control population. Thus, our knowledge on the risk in these patients is scarce, or actually nonexistent.

In both Parkinson's disease and amotrophic lateral sclerosis, single studies have shown that there is no increased risk. The risk in patients with brain tumors and stroke are at present insufficiently documented to make any safe conclusions. Therefore, carefully conducted studies in these disorders are recommended.

Chapter 6

Cancer and Suicide

Cancer is a much feared disease. The course of the disease can be unpredictable and associated with unpleasant treatments such as surgical interventions, chemotherapy, and radiation therapy. Such treatments cause a considerable amount of pain. Cancer victims may suffer from loss of abilities, psychological problems, crisis reaction, and economical changes due to loss of income. The impact on other family members may be tremendous. Furthermore, the fear that the cancer is fatal within a short time exists for a number of cancers, such as lung cancer.

Several studies have examined the relationship between cancer and mental disorders, and an increased risk for mental disorders in cancer patients has been found (Dorpat and Ripley, 1960; Derogatis et al., 1983; Noyes and Kathal, 1986; Plumb and Holland, 1981; Petty and Nayes, 1981; Rodin and Voshart, 1986; Lynch, 1995; Richards, 1994).

Due to the above-mentioned, it would be obvious to expect that among people diagnosed with cancer, *some would choose suicide* to avoid the expected suffering. Another reason for this expectation is the common believe that cancer is identical to a death sentence. Therefore, the afflicted individual wants to take control of the course of the disease.

A number of studies and a few reviews have examined this aspect (Saunders and Valente, 1988; Stenager, Jensen, and Bille-Brahe, 1991; Stiefel, Volkenaandt, and Breitbart, 1989; Perrone, 1993). However, due to methodological problems—among others—the results on cancer and suicide are confusing.

In the literature on cancer and suicide, two completely different methodological types have been used. These types have already been commented on in Chapter 4. The studies are either based on patient registers (Table 6.1) or forensic material (Tables 6.2 and 6.3).

TABLE 6.1. Suicide and Cancer: Epidemiological Studies

Study	Period Year	Sex	Number of suicides	Relative Risk	SMR	Comments
Campbell Connecticut	1959-1962	Male Male	2<55 year 15>55 year	3.6 2.2		suicide risk increased
		Female Female	0<55 year 2>55 year	1.2		small sample, relative risk
			Total =19	3.8		estimated
Farberow et al. California	1959-1966		Total = 40			suicide risk increased, no statistical method used
Louhivouri and Hakama Finland	1965 1960 1966	Male Female	49 14	1.3 (p<0.01) 1.9 (p<0.05)		suicidal risk increased, problems in suicide definition
			Total = 63	1.4		correct statistical method
Fox et al. Connecticut	1940-1969	Male Female	192		2.3 0.9	suicide risk increased correct statistical method
Marshall, Burnett, and Brasure New York	1974-1978	Male Female	112 43	1.6 1.3		suicide risk increased, correct statistical method
			Total = 155			

					suicide risk increased
Olafson Norway	1966-1978	Male Female	117 62 Total = 179		
Allebeck Sweden	1962-1979	Male Female Male Female	645 318 138 44	1.9 1.6 16.0 15.4	suicide risk increased correct statistical method one year after diagnosis
Levi Switzerland	1976-1987	Male Female	39 16 Total = 55 Total = 25	2.76 2.22 3.95	one year after diagnosis
Storm, Christensen, and Jensen Denmark	1971-1986	Male Female Male Female	352 216 115 48	1.5 1.3 2.0 1.4	one year after diagnosis

STUDIES BASED ON PATIENT REGISTERS

In the period from 1959 to 1962 Campell (1966) compared all suicides in Connecticut to the Connecticut Tumor Registry. Twenty-four suicides among the cancer patients were found. The results showed that cancer patients had an increased risk of suicide compared to the background population. The risk was especially increased in older men. However, due to the small number of patients, the results have to be considered with caution.

The frequency of suicides in the period 1959 to 1966 in a somatic hospital in Los Angeles, California, was studied by Farberow and colleagues. Among the cancer patients, 23.4 percent committed suicide. The cancer patients comprised 11.4 percent of all admitted patients in the hospital. The conclusion was that cancer patients had a 12 percent overrepresentation. There were no suicide rates, age distribution, or gender distribution published, which considerably limited the value of the study.

In the years 1955, 1960, and 1965, Louhivouri and Hakama examined 28,847 patients with cancers registered in the Finnish Cancer Registry, and identified sixty-three patients who had committed suicide using violent methods. The suicide risk was calculated, and was determined to be increased in both genders. The study showed that divorced and single cancer patients had a higher risk of suicide than married cancer patients. Patients with a non-localized tumor had a higher risk of suicide than patients with a localized tumor. In a follow-up study, the risk of suicide was shown to be highest within the first five years after the diagnosis was made. In Connecticut, Fox and colleagues in the period from 1940 to 1969 studied all diagnosed cancer patients, a total of 144,530, and found 192 suicides. A comparison to the frequency of suicide in the background population was made. In this comparison, the decade in which the patients were diagnosed, the age of the patient at diagnosing, and the number of years since diagnosing were taken into account. Standardized mortality ratios (SMR) were calculated (see Chapter 3). The SMR was increased in men, but not in women. The risk of suicide was especially increased shortly after the diagnosis was made, which confirmed the result from the study by Louhivouri and Hakama.

Marshall, Burnett, and Brasure (1983) compared all persons in the state of New York in the period from 1974 to 1978 who died due to acute myocardial infarction, motorcycle accidents, or suicide to the New York Cancer Registry. Patients in whom cancer was diagnosed at autopsy were excluded. Information was available on 14,962 men and 7,111 women. An increased risk of suicide in both men and women with cancer was found.

In Norway, Olafsen (1981) registered suicide among cancer patients in the period from 1966 to 1978. A total of 154 from committed suicide. The patients were distributed into three age groups: younger than forty years, forty to fifty-nine years, and more than sixty years of age. Patients older than sixty years had a 2.6 times increased relative risk. Men above sixty years of age had an especially increased risk. Finally, men with cancer in the digestive system (33 percent) and women with breast cancer and ovarian and uterine cancer (70 percent) were at the highest risk of suicide.

Confirming the results by Louhivouri and Hakama (1979) and Fox and colleagues (1982), Olafsen (1981) found the risk of suicide was highest in the first year after the diagnosis was made. A total of 40 percent of the suicides occurred in the first year after diagnosing, and 53.2 percent within the first two years.

One of the most recent studies on cancer and suicide was performed in Sweden in the period 1962 to 1979. Allebeck, Bolund, and Ringbäck (1989) examined 424,127 patients in the Swedish Cancer Registry and found 963 suicides. Based on comparison with the background population, the SMR on the suicide risk was calculated at 1.9 for men and 1.6 for women. In the first year after diagnosing, the risk of suicide in men was increased sixteen times and in women 15.4 times. The risk of suicide decreased with advancing time from the time of diagnosis. When the type of cancer was considered, the suicide risk was highest in patients with cancer in the digestive system and lungs.

In two recent, high-quality studies from a methodological point of view, by Levi, Buillard, and La Vecchia (1991) from Switzerland and Storm, Christensen, and Jensen (1992) from Denmark, the results were confirmed, i.e., the risk of suicide was higher among cancer patients than in the normal population, and the risk was highest in the first year after the diagnosis was made. The Danish study also documented that the risk of suicide has augmented over the years.

As has been documented, agreement exists that the risk of suicide in cancer patients as a group is increased compared to the general population. The size of the risk has varied from 0.9 to 2.2 in women and in men from 1.3 to 3.6. The most convincing results from a statistical point of view agrees on the size of the risk in men (respectively 1.9 and 2.8), but disagrees on the size of the risk in women. The difference can be explained as bias at sampling and registration. Furthermore, the validity of suicide registration varies in many countries. Finally, the size of the studies and the period of data sampling differs, which also may explain differences in the results.

A further point to consider is the fact that the frequency of suicide differs in various populations due to religious, social, and cultural differences. As an example, in the homogenous and ethnically identical population of the Scandinavian countries, the frequency of suicide differs greatly. The frequency is high in Finland and Denmark, lower in Sweden, and lowest in Norway. Such differences may also be reflected in the tendency of cancer patients to choose suicide as a solution in communities with a high frequency of suicide compared to communities with a low frequency.

A further difference may be which deaths are registered as suicide. As an example, Allebeck, Bolund, and Ringbäck (1989) and Fox and colleagues (1982) used the definition of suicide found in the International Classification of Diagnosis (ICD7 and ICD8), while Louhivouri and Hakama (1979) only identified suicides due to *violent* causes, i.e., excluding poisoning. As a consequence of this method of registration, the death of female Finnish cancer patients due to self-poisoning in particular would not be registered.

Studies have shown that women use poison as a method of suicide. Allebeck, Bolund, and Ringbäck determined the rates for women to be 40 percent and for men, 20 percent. However, it is not possible to explain the variance in the risk of suicide among men and women due to differences in registration.

Common to all studies is the notion that the number of suicides probably is underestimated. Suicide is frequently associated with taboo. Therefore, many poisonings in cancer patients will not be registered as suicide, but considered as a natural cause of death in a severely ill person.

STUDIES BASED ON FORENSIC MATERIAL

The studies quoted next are based on forensic studies (see Tables 6.2 and 6.3). In a study from 1955, Sainsbury (1986) claimed that the frequency of cancer among 390 persons who had committed suicide was twenty times higher than in the remaining population. The study, however, provided no statistical documentation for this assertion (See Table 6.2.)

TABLE 6.2. Suicide and Cancer: Autopsy Studies

Study	Period Year	Number of suicides in the study	Number of suicides among cancer patients	Comments
Sainsbury England	1955	390	14	suicide risk increased, no documentation
Dorpat, Ripley Seattle	1957-1958	80	6	suicide risk increased
Whitlock (1978) Brisbane, Australia	1965-1967 1973	273	17 p<0.001	suicide risk increased, the controls are not representative
Hjortsjö Sweden	1972-1973	686	17 male 4 female	suicide risk increased, no documentation
Whitlock (1986) Wales	1968-1972	1,000	32 p<0.001	suicide risk increased
Stensman and Sundqvist-Stensman Sweden	1977-1984	416	13 p<0.001	suicide risk increased
Pollack, and Missliwetz Austria	1967-1976	77	18	no increased suicide risk, very selected material

In a study of eighty suicides, Dorpat and Ripley (1960) found that 7.5 percent had cancer, contrasting 0.43 percent in the background population is Seattle, Washington.

In Brisbane, Australia, in the period from 1965 to 1967 and in 1973, Whitlock (1978) examined 273 suicides in persons who were above fifty years of age and had been examined by autopsy. The suicides were matched on sex and age to persons killed in traffic accidents in the same period. In the suicide group, seventeen persons had cancer, while two had cancer in the control group. The difference was statistically significant. However, the control group was probably not representative of the background population, because cancer patients generally did not drive as frequently as healthy persons.

In Sweden in the period 1972 to 1973, Hjortsjö (1987) studied 686 suicide victims who had been autopsied. Seventeen (4 percent) of all men, and four (1 percent) of all women had cancer. Hjortsjö concluded that this was equivalent to the result in the study by Sainsbury.

Another study by Whitlock (1986) included 1,000 forensically examined suicides in the period from 1968 to 1972 in England and Wales. The study contained information on several somatic disorders. The study found that the frequency of cancer among persons committing suicide was significantly higher compared to the background population. Again in Sweden, Stensman and Sundqvist-Stensman (1988) studied 416 suicides in the period 1977 to 1984, and found that compared to the background population, there was an increased frequency of cancer in persons committing suicide.

In a further study from Sweden, Bolund (1985) in the period from 1973 to 1976 studied ninety-five cancer patients who committed suicide. Based on this material, it was estimated that 1.4 percent of all suicides were committed by cancer patients. However, the purpose of the study was *not* to estimate the frequency of suicide in cancer patients, but to *describe* cancer patients who committed suicide. More than half of the suicides occurred within a year after the diagnosis was made.

In Vienna, Pollack and Missliwetz studied 77 patients who had committed suicide during admittance; eighteen had cancer. Most cancer patients could not be operated on and had severe pain; thus, the patients were strongly selected. The study concluded, that in comparison with the yearly number of cancer deaths, the risk of suicide was one in a thousand, and thus very small.

The next two studies are different from the previous quoted studies in the sense that they are based on consecutive forensic examinations.

In the United States, in a study of 1,300 consecutive forensic autopsies, Murphy (1977) found twenty-two persons with cancer, among whom four had committed suicide. Only two of those patients had cancer diagnosed prior to autopsy. The conclusion was that suicide in association with cancer was a rare occurrence. (See Table 6.3.)

TABLE 6.3. Suicide and Cancer in Consecutive Forensic Studies

Study	Year	Number of forensic autopsies	Number of suicides among cancer patients	Comments
Murphy	1977	1,300	4	no increased suicide risk
Gezelius and Eriksson	1978-1985	7,020	22	no increased suicide risk

In Sweden, Gezelius and Eriksson (1988) examined 7,021 consecutive forensic autopsies, among which 1,060 were suicides. Cancer was found in 2.2 percent of the suicides, and 1 percent of the remaining autopsies. A closer examination revealed that approximately one-third of the suicides were not connected with the cancer. By estimating the number of expected cancer patients among 1,060 suicides, a larger number was expected than was actually found. The study concluded that a more thorough examination was needed in order to prove a possible association between cancer and suicide.

Thus, only three studies reject the idea that cancer patients have an increased risk of suicide compared to the background population (Pollak and Missliwetz, 1979; Murphy, 1977; Gezelius and Eriksson, 1988).

CONCLUSION

From a methodological point of view, based on extensive register studies primarily from Scandinavia and to some extent the United States, an increased risk of suicide in cancer patients as a group has been shown to exist. However, the results are contradictory, regarding the risk in men and women, respectively. This may be explained by differences in study methods, registration, and definition of suicide.

A speculative assumption is that the risk of suicide is higher than has been indicated in the studies because a number of suicides caused by poisoning are not registered. Finally, attention is drawn to the high risk of suicide in the period immediately after the diagnosis is made before the disorder is severely advanced.

Chapter 7

Suicide in Patients
with Other Somatic Disorders

As mentioned in previous chapters, a number of studies have dealt with suicide in patients with somatic diseases other than neurological disorders and cancer (Whitlock, 1986; Wolfersdorf, 1988; Wedler, 1991; Dorpat and Ripley, 1960; Stensman and Sundqvist-Stensman, 1988; Hjortsjö, 1987; Pollak and Missliwetz, 1979; Tuckman, Youngman, and Keizman, 1966; Stewart and Leeds, 1960; Sainsbury, 1955). Mostly, forensic studies have been used in order to enlighten this subject. The studies have shown that between 18 percent and 70 percent of persons committing suicide had a somatic disorder. Methodological problems in study design exist on forensic studies as mentioned in Chapter 4. Despite those methodological problems, the studies indicate that persons with somatic disorders also have an increased risk of suicide.

Wells, Golding, and Burnam (1988; 1989) have studied the association of affective disorders, substance abuse, and anxiety in patients with arthritis, diabetes, heart disease, high blood pressure, and chronic lung condition. It was found that the occurrence of the mentioned mental disorders were increased when compared to a healthy population.

Alcohol and medication abuse, anxiety, and depression are associated with increased risk of suicide, and thus support the hypothesis that an association between suicide and somatic disorder exists.

To be able to prevent suicidal behavior, it is of utmost importance to know which sufferings can cause an increased risk of suicide.

Therefore, the following will deal with our present knowledge on the risk of suicide in patients with heart and lung conditions, disorders or the gastrointestinal canal, kidney conditions, rheumatological disorders, endocrinological disorders, and others.

HEART AND LUNG CONDITIONS

In a review from 1986, Whitlock described the results from a study of 1,000 suicides in England and Wales. In this study, the number of suicides in patients with heart and lung disease did not exceed the expected number. In a study of patients admitted to hospital, Farberow and colleagues (1971) found an increased number of suicides in patients with lung diseases. Shapiro and Waltzer (1980) found an increased number of suicide attempts in patients with lung disorders. None of the quoted studies fulfilled the methodological demands needed in order to determine whether or not there is an increased risk of suicide in persons with lung diseases. No other systematic studies have been performed.

In 1960, Farberow (Farberow et al., 1966) compared persons with heart and lung disorders who committed suicide with persons who did not. He found that those who committed suicide had more emotional problems, and frequently were considered as problem patients by the hospital staff.

Sawyer and colleagues (1983) have explained why patients with lung disorders could be expected to have an increased suicide risk. Frequently, such patients are depressed, anxious, and worried about their condition. Lack of oxygen caused by lung disorders may lead to organic brain syndromes. Reduction in activities of daily living may result in emotional instability. However, Sawyer and colleagues did not examine the frequency of suicide in patients with lung diseases, but rather they only described a single case.

In heart disorders, recent studies on suicide risk have been engaged in estimating whether medication used for reducing the level of cholesterol in the blood (risk factor for developing arteriosclerosis in heart arteries), could induce an increased risk of suicide and other types of violent deaths.

The most comprehensive study was made by Neaton and colleagues in 1992. The study included 350,000 men followed for twelve years. This study found a 1.6 times increased suicide risk in men with a low cholesterol level.

A metaanalysis, i.e., compiling the results of a number of identical studies, by Jacobs and colleagues (1992) reached a similar, though less specific, conclusion. People with low cholesterol level had an increased risk of dying from other reasons than heart disorders, including suicide.

Obviously, a number of uncertainties are involved in such studies. Among others, a number of coexisting factors are not included in the results.

A study published in 1995 by LaRosa did not find any association between low cholesterol level and mortality from other disorders, apart from heart diseases.

Thus, as concluded by Conwell (1995) in his column in *Crisis*, at the present time no studies have definitely documented whether or not there is an association between medically induced reduction of cholesterol level and suicide risk. According to Conwell, this subject is of special interest for those engaged in the care of older patients.

GASTROINTESTINAL DISORDERS

Bowel Disorders

Ulcerative colitis and Crohn's disease are inflammatory disorders of the colon and ileum, respectively. Frequently, young people are afflicted. The disorders result in pains, diarrhea, fatigue, and loss of weight. Usually, the treatment is medication, including among others steroids. One of the side effects of steroid use is an increased risk of psychic instability, such as hypomanic or depressive conditions. In severe cases, surgical removal of parts or the entire colon or ileum may be necessary, resulting in colostomy or ileostomy.

Studies have been made in order to decide whether these disorders are psychosomatic, i.e., psychic conditions that result in somatic disorders. Sheffield and Garney (1976) compared patients with Crohn's disease and controls with other medical disorders without pychosomatic characteristics. Patients with Crohn's disease were more frequently anxious and neurotic than the controls. Therefore, it could be expected that patients with Crohn's disease had an increased risk of suicide.

In line with this expectation, Cooke and colleagues (1980) in a follow-up study found an increased risk of suicide in patients with Crohn's disease. However, a comparison with a control group was not made. Consequently, the results have to be considered with reservation. No other studies have been made estimating the risk of suicide.

In a Norwegian study from 1978, Grüner and colleagues (1987) examined the risk of suicide, risk of mental disorder, and use of psychotropic medication in 178 patients who had experienced a colostomy due to ulcerative colitis. No association between the disorder and risk of suicide or mental disorder was found. The use of psychotropic medication did not differ from the use in the background population.

In 1990 North and colleagues reviewed the literature on ulcerative disorders and mental disorders. Many of the studies on the subject had considerable methodological flaws. In seven methodologically accurate studies, no association was found between ulcerative colitis and mental disorders. Consequently, no increased risk of suicide due to mental instability should be expected in this disorder.

Gastric Disorders

Studies made several years apart have documented an association between alcoholism and the risk of getting peptic ulcer. Alcoholism is also an important risk factor in suicide (Hagnell and Wretmark, 1957; Bergiund, 1986). Logically, an increased risk of suicide could be expected among those suffering from peptic ulcers.

In accordance with this expectation, Whitlock (1986) in his study of 1,000 suicides in England and Wales found an increased risk of suicide in patients with a peptic ulcer. In 1963 both Krause and Westlund had made similar observations. Westlund found the highest risk of suicide in patients subjected to a surgical treatment.

Knop and Fischer (1981) estimated the incidence of suicide in 1,000 patients with a surgical treatment for duodenal ulcer. After an observation period from 21 to 29 years, 13.7 percent of the deceased patients had committed suicide. In men, 12.1 suicides were expected, but fifty-two were found. Among women, seven suicides were found, and 1.3 had been expected. Both differences were statistically significant. Psychiatric morbidity was very high. Among persons who committed suicide, 50 percent were alcoholics. The authors recommended awareness of psychic problems in this group of patients, especially in the phase after surgical treatment.

In a Danish study from 1977 based on 235 deaths in 1,905 patients with a peptic ulcer, Bonnevie did not find an association between peptic ulcer and suicide risk. This study was different from the previous quoted on a number of sociodemographic variables, which may explain the finding.

In another Danish study based on 2,619 patients with peptic ulcer, duodenal ulcer, and dyspepsia, Viskum (1975) found an increased risk of suicide. The patients had also attempted suicide 4 to 11 times more frequently than a control group.

Finally, an English study (Ross et al., 1992) has confirmed the increased risk of suicide in patients with peptic ulcer.

The quoted studies were all done during a time when the standard treatment was surgical. The present treatment is medication with H2-receptor-antagonists, which is much simpler and more efficient. The association of peptic ulcer and alcoholism is still present. However, today one could imagine that the increased suicidal risk was due to alcoholism, and not peptic ulcer per se. Unfortunately, no recent studies can confirm this assumption.

LIVER TRANSPLANT

Liver transplantation is a new treatment, which is supposed to be very strenuous to the patients. The treatment is extremely resource-demanding and the availability of suitable organs is minimal. Therefore, transplantation centers usually have a screening of the mental status of the recipients as a routine, in order to detect contraindications against operation. Possible candidates of liver transplantation could be expected to suffer from depression, anxiety, cognitive dysfunction, and uncertainty regarding the future. The clinical impression is, however, that suicide is a rare occurrence in candidates for liver transplants and that the patients are generally optimistic.

However, in a case report from 1994, Riether and Mahler

describe an increasing number of reports on liver transplant patients attempting or committing suicide. Furthermore, descriptions of patients not following the prescribed treatment are emerging.

In their report, the authors describe four cases of liver transplant patients attempting or committing suicide. They advocate that prior to transplantation, utmost attention should be given to the psychic problems in potential recipients of transplants, and that the patients consecutively receive adequate treatment. The purpose is to secure liver transplants for those patients who have the best opportunities of achieving a good quality of life after the operation. Cooperation between transplantation centers and liaison psychiatrists is recommended.

Due to the small number of transplants performed and the small number of suicides, it is extremely difficult to decide whether or not liver transplant patients have an increased mortality due to suicide.

KIDNEY DISORDERS

Renal transplantation in patients with renal failure is a treatment that has been used for decades in a group of patients who could have an increased risk of suicide.

In 1971 Abram, Moore, and Vestervelt performed a study on suicidal behavior in patients with renal failure. Suicidal behavior was defined as inclusive of the following: (1) suicide, (2) suicide attempt, (3) requesting stop of renal dialysis, and (4) death due to lack of ability or will to carry through renal dialysis. The study included 3,478 renal dialysis patients. A total of 20 patients committed suicide, which meant that the risk of suicide was 100 times that of the normal population, in which the risk was equivalent of 10 per 100,000. The studied population was not matched for sex and age, but in spite of that, the study hinted at an increased risk of suicide in renal dialysis patients.

If deaths due to suicide, stopping treatment, or refusing treatment was included, the risk was increased 400 times compared to the normal population. A total of 5 percent of the dialysis patients exhibited suicidal behavior.

In 1980 Haenel, Brunner, and Battegay, based on a questionnaire sent to renal dialysis and transplantation centers in Switzerland, examined the frequency of suicide among renal dialysis and transplant patients. Furthermore, the frequency of suicide among renal dialysis and transplant patients in Europe was estimated, based on the European Dialysis and Transplant Association Registry.

The study demonstrated that suicide frequently occurs in dialysis patients. In Switzerland, 10 of 574 (1.74 percent) died due to suicide, and 26 of 574 (4.52 percent) due to suicide or refusing treatment. Based on the Swiss suicide rate, it was estimated that the risk of suicide in dialysis patients was increased twenty-five times compared to the normal population. An age and sex standardization was not made.

Also, the European part of the study demonstrated an increased mortality in renal dialysis and transplant patients due to suicide. No major difference in frequency of suicide in renal dialysis and renal transplant patients was found. This was unexpected. An explanation could be that even after a successful transplant, considerable problems may occur, such as side effects due to immunosuppressive treatment. Methodological problems due to the small number of patients may also be part of the explanation.

In accordance with the study on liver transplants, it was recommended that a careful psychiatric evaluation of potential recipients be performed. Similarly, Washer and colleagues (1983) also reported an increased risk of suicide in renal transplant patients, and they recommended a careful psychological follow-up in the patients.

In a letter in *Lancet*, Montandon and Frey (1991) discussed whether or not the choice of immunosuppressive treatment may influence the risk of suicide after renal transplantation.

A study by Burton and colleagues (1986) examined the association of depression and renal failure. They concluded that demographic and psychosocial factors influenced survival more than physiological factors.

In conclusion, the studies have shown that patients with renal failure have an increased risk of suicide. The magnitude of risk is uncertain, partially due to methodological problems in the quoted studies. Evaluation of psychosocial conditions is certainly important in this patient group.

ENDOCRINOLOGICAL DISORDERS

Diabetes Mellitus

The methodological problems discussed in Chapter 4 also have to be kept in mind when we are comparing studies on mortality in diabetics. The authors have used various measures.

The following methods were used in studying diabetics:

1. Mortality ratios (observed deaths/expected deaths)
2. Death rates (deaths/1,000)
3. Percentage (percentage of diabetics who died in one year compared to percentages of those who died in another year from the same cause)
4. Age- and sex-standardized mortality ratios (SMR)

The final method, SMR, has only been used in one published study. The studies are presented in Table 7.1.

In Oslo, Westlund (1969) studied causes of mortality in 3,882 diabetics who were followed from their first discharge after having been diagnosed in the period from 1925 to 1955 and until 1961. He found an increased mortality due to suicide with a mortality ratio of 2.8.

Marks and Krall (1971) reported the principal cause of death in 27,966 deceased diabetics who were treated at the Joslin Clinic between 1897 and 1968. In the period 1897 to 1922, before insulin treatment was established, 0.2 to 0.3 percent of the deaths were due to suicide. In the period 1922 to 1955, 0.4 to 0.7 percent committed suicide, and in the last period to 1968, the percentage was 0.2 to 0.3. No comparison with the general population was made.

In the United States, Goodkin (1975) reported the causes of death among 10,538 diabetics who in the period from 1951 to 1970 applied for life insurance at an American life insurance company. A total of 1,354 died, among whom 4.4 percent died due to accidents or suicide, which was reported to be a greater proportion than in the total population.

In 1977, MacGregor published a follow-up study of fifty diabetic patients diagnosed before the age of thirteen years. Among these patients, forty-four were identified, and seven of these (15 percent)

TABLE 7.1. Suicides in Diabetic Patients: Mortality Studies

Study	Period of Years	Total Number of Deaths	Number of Suicides	Standardized Mortality Ratio (SMR)	Comments
Deckert, Poulsen, and Larsen	1933-1973	173	3%	No SMR	
Joner and Patrick	1973-1988	20		No SMR	
Goodkin	1959-1971	1,354	4.4%	No SMR	
Marks and Krall	1897-1914 1914-1922 1922-1936 1937-1949 1950-1955 1956-1959 1960-1968	326 836 4,157 7,787 5,646 4,205 5,009	0.3% 0.2% 0.7% 0.6% 0.4% 0.2% 0.3%	No SMR or relative risk	Not compared to general population
MacGregor	1950-1975	7	28%	3.4	
Tunbridge	1979	448			Death certificate study Mentions seven deaths of hypogly-cemia which might have been sui-cides
Westlund	1925-1961	2,677			Statistical method correct
Kyvik et al.	1949-1964	168	12%	1.6 2.98 (aged 20 to 24 years)	Statistical method correct

69

had died. Two patients had committed suicide. He compared this result to known suicide statistics in young people, and he calculated a mortality ratio of more than 800. However, this result is most certainly biased because the very small selected study group and no matched control group make statistical analysis unreliable.

Deckert, Poulsen, and Larsen (1978) conducted a follow-up study of 307 patients with diabetes mellitus diagnosed before 1933 who were followed until the end of 1972. Sixty percent of the patients had died, and 3 percent of those deaths were due to suicide. This result, compared to the percentage of death by suicide in the normal population, was not found to be increased.

Joner and Patrick (1991) followed a group of 1,908 diabetic patients between 1973 and 1982. They had onset of diabetes before the age of fifteen years. Twenty died, among whom two were due to suicide.

Tunbridge studied factors contributing to death among young diabetics by reviewing death certificates. The number of suicides was not presented, but among seventeen patients dead due to hypoglycemia, 6 had previously made suicide attempts.

Only one study fulfills the methodological demands necessary for making solid conclusions—a Danish study by Kyvik and colleagues from 1994. The study was comprised of 1,682 male patients with insulin-dependent diabetes mellitus (IDDM). Twelve men committed suicide, and men in the age interval from 20 to 24 years of age had an increased risk of suicide with an SMR of 2.98. The SMR for the whole group was 1.6. Furthermore, the study concluded that the risk of suicide in patients with IDDM might be underestimated because many patients died from unknown causes.

The present review of the literature on suicide risk and diabetes mellitus reveals that only one study has been able to prove an increased risk of suicide among male diabetic patients. Furthermore, a few more studies (Westlund, 1969; MacGregor, 1977) could indicate an increased risk, but only one of these studies has used appropriate methods. A further problem, especially in diabetics, is that suicide statistics may not be reliable. In some cases, death will be registered as a natural cause and not as suicide. Identifying the cause of death in diabetic patients can be difficult, because sudden and unexpected deaths due to hypoglycemia and diabetic coma occur. As pointed out by Tunbridge, some of these deaths may actually be suicides, thus causing a possible underregistration of suicides.

Cushing's Syndrome

In the previously quoted study by Whitlock, he concluded that the number of suicides in patients with endocrinological disorders did not exceed the expected number.

In the literature, case reports on suicide in thyrotoxicosis (Linkowski et al., 1983; Drummond, Lodrick, and Hallstrom, 1984) and Cushing's syndrome exist (Haskett, 1985; Starr, 1952; Taft, Martin, and Melick, 1970), but methodologically sound studies confirming an increased risk of suicide in those endocrinological disorders have not been conducted. Thyrotoxicosis involves an increased level of thyroid hormone and Cushing's syndrome involves an elevated level of adrenocortical hormone. Studies have confirmed that these disorders are associated with an increased risk of mental disorders, which are a known risk factor in suicide (Haskett, 1985; Linkowski et al., 1983).

Regarding disorders of the pituitary gland, no studies on suicide have been performed. Serotonin and its metabolites are neurotransmitters in many areas of the brain, including the pineal gland, where melatonin is produced. Some studies indicate that metabolites from the metabolizing of serotonin measured in the spinal fluid might be associated with an increased risk of suicide (Åsberg, Träskman, and Thoren, 1976).

In conclusion, endocrinological disorders as well as neurotransmitters may be associated with increased risk of suicide. Well-conducted studies on this aspect are much needed.

RHEUMATOLOGICAL AND RELATED DISORDERS

The literature on rhematological disorders and suicide risk has especially concentrated on arthritis and patients who have had amputations. The last group involves studies of World War II soldiers.

Whitlock (1986) did not find any association between arthritis and the risk of suicide, while Dorpat and Ripley (1960), based on their forensic studies, reported a two to three times increased number of suicides in patients with arthritis compared to the expected number, based on the frequency of the disorder in the background population.

Radford, Doll, and Smith (1977) examined the mortality in patients with Becterew's disease, a disorder of the spine involving pain and decreasing flexibility. They compared patients treated with radiotherapy with patients not receiving such therapy. They found that the mortality was increased four times compared to the normal population, and the number of suicides was increased. Only a small number of patients participated, and statistical analysis was not performed.

Shukla and colleagues (1982) examined the frequency of psychiatric disorders in seventy-two patients who had an arm or leg amputated. Almost two-thirds had suffered from depression, anxiety, insomnia, loss of appetite, suicide ideation, and psychotic behavior.

Bakalim (1969) studied 4,738 amputees from the Finnish-Soviet War, and found an increased risk of suicide compared to the normal male population. The risk of suicide was increased 37.3 percent, and was even higher in the youngest victims of war.

It is debatable whether it is the loss of an arm or leg alone, or the circumstances of participating in war and being a war casualty, that influence the risk of suicide. The last suggestion seems to be the most reasonable.

Hrubec and Ryder (1979) also have examined the risk of suicide in war amputees hospitalized during 1944 to 1945 in the United States. The study did not find a statistical excess of suicides in the amputee group, but the group studied had a relative risk of 5.1 for suicide by poisoning.

Since these studies were performed, treatment possibilities have improved, but whether or not this has changed the risk of suicide has not been studied.

TINNITUS

Tinnitus involves a continuous unpleasant sound in the ear. Musicians and persons subjected to noise are often afflicted. The disorder is associated with an increased risk of depression. Harrop-Griffith and colleagues (1987) found that the lifetime prevalence of depression was 62 percent in patients with tinnitus compared to 21 percent in a control group. Erlandson and Archer (1994) also found an increased risk of depression in patients with tinnitus.

In the period from March 1990 to April 1991, four committed suicide among the patients with tinnitus at the audiology clinics in Cardiff, Wales. Due to these incidences, Lewis, Stephens, and McKenna (1994) initiated a study on tinnitus and suicidal behavior. They contacted fifty audiology clinics in the United Kingdom, Europe, North America, Australia, and Japan and asked for systematically collected information on patients with tinnitus who had committed suicide.

They collected information on twenty-eight suicides. The suicides occurred especially among men, older persons, and those who were socially isolated. A high percentage of mental disorders (94 percent) was found among patients committing suicide, especially depression (70 percent), which was more than usually found among patients with tinnitus. Five of the patients had at least at one occasion attempted suicide. Forty percent of the suicides were committed within the first year after onset of the disorder, and 50 percent within the first two years after onset. The results of this study indicated that tinnitus was an important risk factor, compared to the other suicide risk factors.

Using a crude comparison, the authors determined that the risk of suicide was increased in patients with tinnitus compared to the background population. As indicated previously, such comparisons are connected with serious risk of bias.

AIDS

AIDS has spread vigorously all over the world. Efficient treatments are still not available. Therefore, considerations of the suicide risk among AIDS patients have emerged.

Shortly after the illness had been recognized, Marzuk and colleagues in 1988 published a study from New York, indicating that the risk of suicide in men suffering from AIDS was thirty-six times higher than in healthy men (1988). This increased risk was confirmed by Kizer and colleagues in 1988 in a study from California. Using death certificates, they found that the risk of suicide for men in the age-interval 20 to 39 years of age with AIDS was increased twenty-one times (1988).

The ways health care professionals—as well as the general public—treat patients with AIDS has changed since the first studies were conducted, which positively may have influenced the risk of suicide. The possibilities of treatment have improved in the sense that patients may live longer with the disorder now. In some communities, social stigmatizing may have decreased as a better understanding of the illness has developed.

In 1992, Coté, Biggar, and Dannenberg published a study on all deaths due to suicide in forty-five states in the United States from 1987 to 1989. They found that the risk of suicide in patients with AIDS was 7.4 times higher than in the background population. The risk had been decreasing during the observation period. The authors interpreted this as an indication of the improved treatment possibities. However, one obvious bias, which was not considered, was the risk that both suicide and AIDS were underestimated.

Finally, a study has been conducted with the aim of evaluating whether or not a positive test of HIV is associated with an increased risk of suicide (Perry, Jacobsberg, and Fishman, 1990). The study demonstrated that both HIV-positive and HIV-negative persons had suicidal thoughts in the test period, but the thoughts vanished within a two-month period. Among both seropositive and seronegative tested, 5 percent continuously had suicidal thoughts. They also showed signs of depression.

In conclusion, AIDS has been associated with increased risk of suicide, but methodological problems also exist in these studies.

CONCLUSION

The review of the literature on somatic disorders and suicide risk has shown that probably a number of disorders are associated with an increased risk of suicide. Most studies were based on case reports, and rarely on major methodologically sound surveys. A rare exception is the study on the risk of suicide in diabetics (Kyvik et al., 1994). Furthermore, most studies are old; therefore, we do not know if improvements in treatment are reflected in the risk of suicide.

As we have seen in the studies of neurological disorders and cancer, the risk of suicide was associated with psychological and social problems. We would expect the same tendency in other somatic disorders. How-ever, no one has shown interest in studying similar problems in frequently met disorders, such as heart disease, lung disorders, arthritis, and endocrinological disorders. Both from the patients' point of view and for scientific reasons, such studies are very much needed.

Despite that the idea that illness should be considered as a biological, psychological, and social process has spread, it is surprising that this has not resulted in studies on suicidal behavior. Suicidal behavior can be considered as the final consequence of psychological, biologial, and social problems in the patient.

Chapter 8

Suicide Attempts
and Somatic Disorders

The association of somatic disorder and suicide attempt has not been as carefully examined as the association of somatic disorder and suicide.

Several types of study designs are found. Generally, the problems connected with the validity of the studies are even greater in studies on suicide attempt than they are in studies on suicide. One of the reasons is that the definition of suicide attempt differs in the various studies. Some studies, especially the most recent (Bille-Brahe, 1993), have used the World Health Organization's (1986) definition:

> An act with nonfatal outcome, in which an individual deliberately initiates a nonhabitual behavior, that without intervention of others, will cause self-harm, or deliberately ingests a substance in excess of the prescribed or generally recognized therapeutic dosage, and which is aimed at realizing changes which he/she desired via the actual or expected physical consequences.

Other studies have only used poisoning as defining a suicide attempt. Finally, some studies have used an even more rigorous definition than found in the WHO definition. This includes the demand that the act was deliberate with a suicide intention, i.e., a failed suicide.

Methodologically, a number of designs have been used in the available studies.

1. The frequency of somatic disorders in suicide attempters.
2. Follow-up studies on suicide attempters. The risk of repetition of suicidal behavior in suicide attempters with somatic disorders is estimated.
3. Studies in defined groups of patients. The frequency of suicide is estimated.
4. Studies of defined groups of patients with or without suicide attempt compared to a control group. The purpose is to estimate whether or not a specific group of patients has an increased risk of suicide.

Finally, a heterogeneous literature exists on patients with certain disorders, such as diabetes mellitus, who have attempted suicide.

The following will concentrate on studies on the frequency of somatic disorders among suicide attempters (type 1), follow-up studies (type 2), and studies on the risk of suicide attempt in certain somatic disorders (types 3 and 4).

THE FREQUENCY OF SOMATIC DISORDERS AMONG SUICIDE ATTEMPTERS AND IN FOLLOW-UP STUDIES

In 1980 Nielsen, Wang, and Bille-Brahe (1990) examined 207 suicide attempters admitted to a Danish psychiatric ward. A total of 71 (35 percent) among the 207 patients had a chronic somatic disorder. A chronic somatic disorder was defined as follows: "A disease hampering the patient's daily life, i.e., if the patient has to take analgesics constantly or is to some degree disabled."

The most frequently occurring disorders in the study by Nielsen and colleagues were neurological disorders, gastrointestinal disorders such as gastric ulcers, and rheumatological disorders—mainly benign chronic disorders. A total of twenty-five (13 percent) of the suicide attempters had chronic pain.

The study followed the patients for five years, and the number of suicides and suicide attempts was registered. Suicide attempters with somatic disorders showed an increased risk of suicide. The risk was twice that found in the control group comprised of suicide attempters without a somatic disorder. In his thesis, Nielsen (1994) made a model on risk factors for repetitive suicidal behavior. Based on the previous study, chronic somatic disorder is an important risk factor in this model.

In two studies from Germany, 27 percent and 30 percent of the suicide attempters were shown to suffer from a somatic disorder (Dietzfelbinger et al., 1991; Wedler, 1991). The patients were selected from somatic wards. Comparison for age distribution was impossible because no mean values for age were given. In a recent Swedish study by Öjehagen, Regnell, and Träskman-Bendz (1991), patients admitted to an intensive care unit following a suicide attempt were studied. Approximately half of them were found to suffer from a somatic disorder.

In 1989 Stenager and colleagues (1992) studied 195 suicide attempters treated in a psychiatric ward after the attempt. The study included both admitted patients and outpatients. In this population, forty-three (22 percent) had a chronic somatic disorder, i.e., substantially fewer patients than in the previously quoted Danish study by Nielsen. The study comprised more patients treated as outpatients in the emergency room, which may partially explain the difference found, especially because the definition of a somatic disorder was identical in the two studies. After a one-year follow-up, no association was found between somatic disorders and repetitive suicide attempts (Stenager and Benjaminsen, 1991).

In 1990 Stenager (1992) interviewed a total of 139 suicide attempters admitted to a psychiatric ward after the attempt. The occurrence of somatic disorders was thoroughly evaluated (Stenager, Stenager, and Jensen, 1994). A total of seventy-two (52 percent) of the suicide attempters had a chronic somatic disorder, and twenty-nine (21 percent) used analgesics on a daily basis due to pain, and a further twenty-four (17 percent) used analgesics weekly. The most frequently occurring disorders in this study were rheumatological disorders (50 percent), neurological disorders (22 percent), cardiovascular disorders (15 percent), and gastrointestinal disorders (19 percent). Several patients had more than one disorder. Complaints concerning pain were distributed as follows: headache, seventeen patients (50 percent); arthralgia, nine patients (31 percent); muscle pain, eleven patients (38 percent); low back pain, nine patients (31 percent); and gastrointestinal pain, six patients (14 percent).

The patients with a somatic disorder were compared to patients without such a disorder. Patients with somatic disorders were characterized by the following: they were older and more frequently had daily pains, suffered from psychosis, and had a crisis reaction.

The patients were followed for one year, and repeated suicide attempters were compared with nonrepeaters for the presence of somatic disorders, daily or intermittent pain, and psychiatric diagnosis.

A tendency was seen that patients with a somatic disorder were at lower risk of repetition of suicide attempt. The results were stratified for the presence of depression. Patients with a somatic disease alone seemed to be less at risk for repetition of suicide attempt. No statistically significant difference was found for daily or intermittent pain, somatic disease with pain, or psychiatric diagnosis even when stratified for depression.

On the basis of these studies, it could therefore be expected that between 30 percent and 50 percent of all suicide attempters suffer from a somatic disorder. The number will depend on how the patients are selected, and whether information is obtained by interview or by use of case sheets. Furthermore, the definition used for the suicide attempt is important. Finally, the studies show that physicians treating suicide attempters should be aware of somatic problems.

In a short follow-up period, no association has been found between somatic disorder and repetitive suicidal behavior, contrasting the association found after a five-year follow-up period.

COMPARISON OF SUICIDE ATTEMPTERS AND CONTROL GROUPS

Kontaxakis and colleagues (1988) have compared suicide attempters with concurrent psychiatric and somatic disorder and suicide attempters with a psychiatric disorder alone. They found that suicide attempters suffering from both a somatic and psychiatric disorder were older, more often suffered from an organic psychotic disorder or affective disorder, and more frequently used violent methods in the suicide attempt. The most frequent somatic disorders found in the study were neurological disorders, cardiovascular disorders, and cancer.

Suicide Attempts and Migraine

Breslau, Davis, and Andreski (1991) published a very carefully conducted study on the risk of suicide attempt in migraine patients. Among 1,200 randomly selected twenty-one to thirty-year-old patients, 1,007 participated in a structured interview on headache and migraine. Migraine patients were identified according to defined criteria and compared to nonmigraine patients regarding suicide attempts. The odds ratio for suicide attempt in patients with migraine with aura (warning symptoms of migraine attack) compared to nonmigraine patients was 3.0, i.e., migraine patients have a three times increased risk of a suicide attempt. In a statistical logistic regression model, the results were controlled for depression, others psychiatric disorders, and gender. The final conclusion was that migraine patients had an increased risk of attempting suicide compared to nonmigraine patients.

Suicide Attempts and Epilepsy

Hawton (1987) studied the frequency of epilepsy among patients admitted after a suicide attempt in a two-year period. Based on the prevalence of epilepsy in the background population, the number of suicide attempts in patients with epilepsy was increased five times. Compared to the background population, patients with epilepsy more frequently had received psychiatric treatment, and had made more suicide attempts.

Mendez and colleagues (1989) compared suicide attempters with epilepsy with suicide attempters without epilepsy. They found that patients with epilepsy more frequently had borderline personality disorders, psychotic disorders, and previous suicide attempts.

Suicidal Thoughts and Psoriasis

In an American investigation, Gupta and colleagues (1993) studied the frequency of suicidal thoughts among patients with psoriasis in a dermatological ward, using a self-rating questionnaire. A total of 1,217 patients participated in the study, and a little less than 10 percent expressed death wishes, and 5.5 percent reported suicidal thoughts at the time of participation. Patients with suicidal thoughts were characterized by a higher score (more depressed) on a depression rating scale, and the severity of their disorder was worse compared to patients without suicidal thoughts. An association was found between depression and self-rated experience of the severity of the disorder.

The study demonstrated that even in relatively benign disorders, suicidal thoughts occur. A weakness in this study is the lack of a control group. In the healthy population, a number of depressive moods and suicidal thoughts also occur.

Suicide Attempts and Diabetes Mellitus

The literature is mostly based on case reports concerning specific groups of patients. The studies examined several areas, including insulin overdoses and hypoglycemic episodes, as well as suicide attempts in diabetics.

Insulin Overdoses and Hypoglycemic Episodes

In 1983 Kaminer and Robbins reviewed the literature on insulin overdose. They found 17 suicides and 80 attempted suicides in the literature, and they discussed various aspects of the reported cases. The sex ratio was 1:1, 40 were repeated suicide attempts, and the age distribution among the attempters was even.

In a paper from 1971 on problems in hypoglycemia, Wolff states that suicide and suicide attempts by overdose of insulin are rare. Wolff explains this by the fact that few have easy access to insulin, and they probably know that it is not a reliable medication for suicide. Gale (1980), as a contrast, claims that suicidal overdoses of insulin are not uncommon. In a study of hypoglycemic episodes in an emergency ward in Nottingham, 4 of 204 episodes were suicide attempts.

Case Reports

In the 1960s and 1970s in France, suicide by insulin caused great interest. Several case reports and studies were reviewed, and Bourgeois and Dufourg (1967), Bourgeois (1974), and Chalier (1969) concluded that suicide and suicide attempts in diabetics were uncommon. Nonetheless, they stressed the importance of being aware of the psychological state of diabetic patients.

From Houston, Texas in 1985, Arem and Zogbi reported eight attempted suicides by overdosing on insulin. They also reviewed the literature on suicide by insulin, which was sparse. They were surprised to have found eight cases in their hospital, despite the paucity of case reports in the world literature, and concluded that the problem was more common than previously supposed. Among the eight attempters, seven had depressive symptoms or other psychiatric disorders before the suicide attempt.

Suicide Attempts in Diabetic Patients

In 1983, Jefferys and Volans reported a prospective study on self-poisoning in diabetic patients referred to the National Poisons Information Service in London in the period 1978 to 1979. In the two-year period, 386 diabetic patients were reported. Hypoglycemic medication was used by 64 patients. The remaining patients had used other medications (psychotropic and hypnotic) or household products. Among those using hypoglycemic medication, ten died due to anoxic brain damage. The authors concluded that self-poisoning was common among diabetic patients and suggested toxicological screening in patients with prolonged keto-acedotic coma.

In a paper on social and psychological rehabilitation of diabetic patients, Simons and Schilling (1974) examined the quality of life in 209 patients who had received kidney transplants, among whom 41 were diabetic. The authors tried to document the extent of suicidal behavior that the patients presented to the medical staff. Suicidal behavior was seen in 10 percent of the diabetic patients, and the authors suggested that psychiatric help would be advisable to vulnerable diabetic patients.

In conclusion, the problem of attempted suicide in diabetics has only been examined in a few studies. Two studies (Arem and Zogbi, 1985; Jeffreys and Volans, 1983) concluded that suicide attempts in diabetics were more common than expected, and toxicological screening in prolonged keto-acedotic coma was recommended.

CONCLUSION

This review has shown that a large group of suicide attempters suffer from somatic disorders and pains that affect their daily life and increase their vulnerability. It is important that the physician who may be consulted by the suicide attempter prior to the act is aware that a combination of psychological and social strain, depressive symptoms, a somatic disorder, and pain may precipitate suicidal behavior. Stenager and Jensen (1994) have documented that in particular patients with depression and pain consult their general practitioner prior to a suicide attempt more often than other attempters.

It has been shown that many somatic disorders involve an increased risk of depression, particularly in the case of neurological disorders. In such cases, it is difficult to determine whether the depression is caused by organic or psychological factors (Stenager, Knudsen, and Jensen, 1990; Schiffer, 1990).

The relatively large number of suicide attempters suffering from a neurological disorder, depressive disease, and pain prompts the question whether biological markers, i.e., serotonin, can affect their condition. Previously, it has been mentioned that a low level of the serotonin metabolite HIAA indicates a risk factor in suicidal behavior (Åsberg, Nordstrøm, and Träskman-Bendz, 1986). Furthermore, high serotonin levels alleviate certain kinds of depression and reduce perception of pain, especially chronic pain (Hendler, 1984). A number of antidepressants that block serotonin re-uptake have been found to be very useful in the treatment of mixed states of pain and depression.

Suicide attempters with a somatic disorder but no concurrent depressive disorder seem to have been at a lower risk of repetition of suicide attempt during the one-year follow-up period. A suicide attempt may be an attempt to gain access to health services, be examined by a doctor, and receive treatment for a somatic disorder, and thereby help solve other life problems that could lessen the impact of a poor physical condition. Furthermore, some of the somatic problems could be due to a psychosomatic disorder, such as headache, gastrointestinal pain, and other pain conditions.

One of the studies (Stenager, Stenager, and Jensen, 1994) found an increased risk of suicidal behavior in older patients with painful somatic disorders, which tends to confirm previous indications that depression and somatic disorders are important risk factors in suicide (Nielsen, 1994). The reasons could be as follows:

1. The presence of depression in patients in pain was not recognized, and consequently treatment was inadequate.
2. The somatic disorder was not diagnosed, nor was appropriate treatment initiated.
3. In spite of adequate intervention, some patients cannot be helped and will in any case choose suicide as a way of escaping their situation.

An important task for the physician in suicide prevention is to secure the patient an optimal diagnostic and treatment procedure, if the condition is such that it can be treated. This aspect will be discussed further in the final chapter.

Chapter 9

Pain and Suicidal Behavior

Complaints of pains and chronic pain conditions are frequently met among the general population. In a Canadian study, Crook, Rideout, and Brown (1984) tried to estimate the number of pain complaints in a group of 500 persons in the last fourteen days prior to the study. They found that 116 per 1,000 of the men and 145 per 1,000 of the women had lasting pain within the last fourteen days. The frequency of lasting pain complaints was more than twice the frequency of intermittent pain complaints. More women than men had pain complaints, and the frequency of complaints increased with increasing age. Low back pain, pain in arms and legs, and headache were the most frequent pain complaints. A Danish study (Andersen and Worm-Pedersen, 1987) has confirmed the high prevalence of pains in a Danish population. In this study, 30 percent had pains, among which 17 percent were acute pains.

A study by Kotarba (1983) has estimated that 40 million Americans have a chronic pain condition. Kotarba defines chronic pain as a condition that cannot be suppressed medically.

Based on the knowledge of how devastating a chronic pain condition can be for the individual patient, it is obvious that suicide frequency increases in patients. In the literature reviews in the previous chapters, a number of disorders associated with an increased risk of suicide were documented, including chronic pains such as cancers, certain neurological conditions such as multiple sclerosis, traumatic brain damage, spinal cord lesions, migraine, and diabetic neuropathy. Furthermore, a number of conditions in which the risk of suicide was not properly examined, such as gastrointestinal disorders and rheumatological disorders, were associated with pain conditions.

Despite this knowledge, no studies have examined specifically whether or not patients with chronic pain have an increased risk of suicide. Most studies dealing with this problem—and there are actually a few—are based on case reports. However, a number of questions and problems are associated with studies on pain and suicidal behavior:

- Why is it obvious to assume that pain conditions are associated with increased risk of suicide?
- Are pain conditions and psychic disorders associated?
- What methodological problems are associated with the conduction of such studies?

These problems will be discussed in the following.

WHY IS IT OBVIOUS TO ASSUME THAT PAIN CONDITIONS ARE ASSOCIATED WITH AN INCREASED SUICIDE RISK?

Suicide can be conceived as the final solution to a human being living an unbearable life. A number of causes may contribute to the feeling that life is unbearable, such as social problems; relationships problems with close relatives, colleagues, and friends; or lack of a relationship, which leads to isolation. Problems can be caused by the abuse of alcohol, medication, or drugs. In other cases, human beings are suffering from severe mental disorders such as depression or schizophrenia, and they experience the psychic pain associated with these conditions. Finally, a large number of people have severe somatic conditions that may result in loss of working capacity, limitations of daily life activities, social isolation, psychological problems, psychiatric disorders such as anxiety or depression, and a severe and intractable pain condition.

In some instances, a physiological explanation for the pain is impossible to find, as in some patients with low back pain, fibromyalgia, whiplash pain, unspecified chronic headache, and uncharacteristic aching in the arms and legs. People with such conditions are in an even worse condition than those who have been told an organic explanation for their pain because the former frequently encounter a skeptical attitude from family, friends, and medical and social service professionals. Such skepticism, combined with an impairment, results in a very difficult situation for the patient.

The previously mentioned conditions can lead to a state the nestor of suicidology, Edwin Schneidman, has termed *psychache*. In a commentary, Schneidman (1993) described suicide as a psychache. He found the following six points of importance in the understanding of suicide.

1. The explanation of suicide in humankind is the same as the explanation of suicide of any particular human.
2. Suicides are multidimensional, multifaceted, and multidisciplinary containing concomitant biological, sociological, psychological, epidemiological, and philosophical elements.
3. The key element in every suicide is psychological pain, or psychache. No psychache, no suicide.
4. Individuals have different thresholds for enduring or tolerating pain.
5. In every suicide, the psychological pain is created and fueled by frustrated psychological needs.
6. In an individual, there are psychological needs with which the person lives and psychological needs whose frustration cannot be tolerated. These two kinds of needs are consistent with each other, although not necessarily the same as each other. From the point of view of treatment, it is of importance to be aware of the patient's psychological needs because changes of those needs will change the condition of the patient from suicidal to nonsuicidal.

From the Schneidman theory of the understanding of suicide, it would be assumed that the border between psychological pain and physical pain is blurred in human beings who suffer pain both with and without documented somatic causes. Thus, a pain condition can be one of several reasons why life becomes unbearable. To whom this will happen, and how frequently physical pain is the main cause, we do not know.

THE ASSOCIATION OF PAIN CONDITIONS AND MENTAL DISORDERS

Several studies have been conducted in order to clarify the association of mental disorders and chronic pain conditions. Dufton tried to study the association of pain, emotional functioning, and cognitive insufficiency (1989). He found an association between the tendency of making cognitive errors and emotional difficulties, but this association was not related to pain variables. Dufton suggested several explanations among others that cognitive and affective dysfunction are associated circularly, and that an increased occurrence of cognitive problems can predispose patients with pain to have succeeding affective problems.

In 1984, Roy, Thomas, and Matas reviewed the literature on the association of chronic pain and depression. They found that such an association was hard to prove, partially due to methodological problems. They concluded that chronic pain and depression were not equivalent; chronic pain was not primarily a psychic condition.

Hendler (1985) and Blumer and Heilbronn (1982) have examined if depression could be the cause of chronic pain, or if chronic pain could be a variant of depression. Both studies concluded that the association was extremely complex, and that the methodological problems met were considerable.

Fishbain and colleagues (1986) have used the DSM-III psychiatric diagnostic criteria to describe the psychiatric disorders in patients with chronic pain conditions. According to these criteria, 58.4 percent of the patients had personality disorders, almost 40 percent conversion disorders, and less than 5 percent other somatoform disorders. More than 60 percent had anxiety and panic disorders, and almost 60 percent depressive disorders. Finally, 15 percent had abuse problems. The authors concluded that DSM-III diagnostic criteria with certain limitations could be used to describe mental problems in patients with chronic pain. Based on this study, mental problems were frequently occurring in chronic pain patients.

Finally, Romano and Turner (1985) found in their review that the frequency of depression was higher in patients with chronic pain than in the background population and in patients with other somatic disorders. However, due to a lack of well-conducted controlled studies, it could not be concluded that depressive disorders were more frequent among patients with pain. In some studies, a higher frequency of headache in depressed patients was found, but methodological problems excluded a definite conclusion.

In some studies, approximately 50 percent of the patients with chronic pain and depression developed the two sufferings simultaneously, and 40 percent were depressed some time after the onset of pain. This indicated the existence of at least two subgroups of patients.

This could also indicate that the coexistence of pain and depression was the final presentation of a medical condition.

METHODOLOGICAL PROBLEMS

In their review, Romano and Turner described methodological problems associated with studies on the relation between pain and depression. The problems are frequently encountered when studying the association between pain and suicidal behavior. Therefore, they will be described briefly.

Assessment of Pain and Depression

There are problems associated with the validity and reliability in the diagnosis of both depression and pain. Obviously, this is important in selection of patients and comparisons of results. The frequency of the conditions depend on the diagnostic criteria used.

Selection of Patients

Representative groups of patients both regarding depression and pain are difficult to select. The patients can be selected from different categories of disorders and from various treatment institutions, such as psychiatric wards, outpatients clinics, pain clinics, private practitioners, etc. Due to this variation in selection, comparison of the groups is difficult.

Control Groups

Control groups are necessary in order to be able to estimate the prevalence of the disorders. In their papers, Hendler (1985) and

Blumer and Heilbronn (1982) discuss theories on the classification of pain conditions and the interpretation of such theories. Adler and colleagues (1989) have discussed problems regarding definition of pain. Such discussions are beyond the scope of this book. Interested readers should consult the papers.

STUDIES ON SUICIDAL BEHAVIOR AND PAIN

As previously mentioned, only a few studies exist on pain and suicidal behavior.

In a case report, Bebbington (1976) described two patients with monosymptomatic hypochondriac pain in the eyes who had committed suicide. Kotarba described a patient with chronic pain secondary to rheumatic arthritis, who committed suicide due to acute demoralization. The patient received treatment, but after repetitive treatment failure and reoccurrence of pain, he was increasingly pessimistic regarding his situation. In despair due to the lack of possibilities for a cure, he felt demoralized, hopeless, and depressed, and finally committed suicide.

Fishbain and colleagues (1986) studied suicidal behavior and pain, and concluded that it is important to be able to identify high-risk patients in order to prevent suicide. In their pain clinic, after an unsystematic telephone interview follow-up, they identified three patients with pain who committed suicide. Based on the number of patients with pain and the three suicides, they have tried to estimate the risk of suicide compared to the background population in the United States. Based on this calculation, they found that the risk of suicide in a population of pain patients was increased significantly compared to the background population. Furthermore, they compared the population of pain patients with a population of psychiatric patients, and estimated that pain patients had a lower risk of suicide than psychiatric patients.

As discussed by the authors, considerable problems are found in this study.

1. A psychological autopsy has not been performed. Consequently, it is not known if pain was the cause of suicide.
2. A systematic follow-up was not performed. Therefore, the frequency of suicide may have been higher.

3. Statistically, three suicides could have been incidental.
4. Statistically, it is very problematic to compare three suicides with the risk of suicide in the whole population.
5. The population is narrowly selected.

Despite the numerous methodological problems, the study may indicate that an association between pain and suicidal behavior exists. Therefore, it is recommended that further studies are performed (Fishbain, 1995; Stenager and Stenager, 1995).

Israel Orbach (1994) has also dealt with pain and suicide. He did not report case reports or studies, but based on the literature, he tried to make a theoretical model of the association of dissociative conditions, pain, and suicide. Orbach starts with persons subjected to previous traumatic experience, including extreme repulsion both mentally and physically, leading gradually to bodily indifference demonstrated by physical insensitivity and apathy, eventually resulting in no registration of pain. At onset, stress can protect, but continued stress may result in bodily dissociation and increased risk of self-destructive behavior. Orbach recommended further studies of this topic in order to understand suicidal behavior and thereby improve prevention and treatment.

Livengood and Parris (1992), based on their experience with chronic pain patients, suggest that screening tools for psychiatric disorders be used in chronic pain patients. If suicidal thoughts are found in the screening, a scale of suicidal intention is recommended and then psychiatric evaluation and treatment started.

Before such a routine screening is started, increased knowledge on the risk of suicidal behavior in pain patients would be valuable. This would provide a better basis from which to start such an initiative.

Based on the reported studies, it is not possible to conclude whether or not an association of pain and suicidal behavior exist, but the likelihood of such an association is high. However, a valid method of examining such an association is even more difficult to construct than in studies on suicidal behavior and defined somatic disorders. The reason is the problems connected with validating pain conditions. Should the study only include patients with organic pains in well-defined conditions? Should patients with pain without a well-established organic cause be included? How should pain be defined? How should pain be measured? How should representative and comparable populations be established? How should psychic manifestations involving pain be separated from organic pain? Which tools should be used? The problems are also numerous if standard statistical and epidemiological methods are used.

A possible solution to the many methodological problems in studies concerning suicidal behavior and pain would be having the problems carefully described in qualitative studies. Psychological autopsies could also be used. Thus, defined groups of patients could emerge. Another possibility is to study the frequency of chronic pain in defined groups of patients with an established increased risk of suicide (Stenager, Stenager, and Jensen, 1994). In this respect, Breitbart (1990) already has described severe pain conditions as a cofactor involved in the increased risk of suicide in cancer patients. Obviously, this is an area needing much more research.

Chapter 10

General Aspects of Suicidal Behavior, Pain, and Somatic Disorders

SUICIDAL RISK AND SOMATIC DISORDERS

The review of the literature on suicidal risk in this book has shown that not only patients with mental disorders but also patients with somatic disorders and pain have an increased risk of suicide. Probably, a considerable comorbidity between somatic and mental disorders exists in patients who commit or attempt suicide. However, methodologically sound studies using the background population as a control have concluded that the somatic disorder alone is responsible for an increased risk of suicide.

The review has also demonstrated that the risk of suicide has thoroughly been studied in a number of disorders, such as neurological diseases and cancer, while the knowledge on this association in many frequently occurring disorders, such as heart and lung diseases, is sparse or nonexistent. Furthermore, information on pain and suicidal risk is extremely sparse, which to some extent can be explained by considerable methodological problems in studying this aspect.

Genetic disorders present a special ethical problem regarding risk of suicide, if they can be diagnosed years before onset of the disease, as demonstrated in Huntington's chorea. As genetic technology is advancing rapidly, further knowledge about these disorders and the related suicide risk is much needed.

Advanced medical technology and treatment possibilities were supposed to improve quality of life and consequently reduce the risk of suicide. The suicides in liver and renal transplant patients demonstrate that the situation is more complicated than had been expected. Therefore, similar studies are needed in cardiac, lung, and bone marrow transplant patients.

Similarly, it is astonishing that in the most frequently occurring disorders such as ischaemic heart disease, bronchitis, and asthma, no one has studied the risk of suicide because these sufferings result in considerable reduction of life quality and cause considerable pain and impairment. The onset is often in periods during which the patients are still working, and thus may result in loss of income, perhaps with disablement pension, social, and economic consequences. The review has demonstrated that disorders afflicting younger persons, such as multiple sclerosis, diabetes mellitus, and epilepsy, result in an increased risk of suicide, especially among the youngest sufferers. Thus, diseases affecting young and middle-aged persons are relevant to study in this context.

SUICIDAL RISK AS A MEASURE
OF LIFE QUALITY AND COPING ABILITY

Estimating the risk of suicide in a certain disease could be expected to be easily measurable based on whether or not this disorder results in a reduced quality of life and whether or not the patients succeed in coping with the disorder. Furthermore, the quality of the postdiagnostic psychosocial treatment in various geographic areas is indicated by the differing suicide risks for specific disorders.

In one Danish study (Stenager, Koch-Henriksen, and Stenager, 1996), a lower risk of suicide was found in an area with a long-standing tradition for outpatient treatment of a chronic disorder compared to areas with no such options.

The estimation of the risk of suicide is a relatively simple epidemiological measure, especially in frequently occurring disorders, if proper registration of patients and national registration of causes of death exist. Thus, the measure can be determined in at least the Scandinavian countries.

Finally, the standard tests of life quality are usually comprehensive, time-consuming, and limited to a small number of patients in a short time interval, while estimation of risk of suicide enables a continuous survey in large groups of patients in long time intervals after diagnosing.

PREVENTION OF SUICIDAL BEHAVIOR IN PATIENTS WITH SOMATIC DISORDERS

Suppose a clinician knows that a certain disease is associated with an increased risk of suicide. How should this situation be handled? In order to answer this question, we have to consider the following points:

1. What signals indicating risk of suicide are present?
2. How is suicide prevented?
3. Should suicide always be prevented?
4. What questions should be asked to a patient at risk of suicide?

What Signals Indicating Risk of Suicide Are Present?

When the clinician meets a patient, he or she should be aware of a number of signals that may indicate an increased risk of suicide in this patient.

Does the Patient Have a Mental Disorder?

Depression and anxiety disorders are associated with an increased risk of suicide, as discussed in Chapter 3. The patient may have an organic psychosyndrome, which could be caused by metastases in a cancer patient or could be medically induced, for example, by steroids. The syndrome could indicate an increased risk of suicide. Psychosis for other reasons involves increased risk as well.

Has the Patient Previously Attempted Suicide?

Previous suicide attempt or suicidal behavior in the family indicate an increased risk.

Does the Patient Express Suicidal Thoughts?

Such thoughts should not be neglected.

Does the Patient Feel That Life Is Hopeless?

Hopelessness in addition to loss of abilities and fear of a painful death could be a contributing cause of suicide. The feeling of hopelessness in patients admitted after a suicide attempt can be an important predictor of a future suicide.

Does the Patient Have Pain?

Reports on pain are important. Bolund (1985a,b) found that 85 percent of patients with cancer who committed suicide had severe pain. Other chronic disorders with increased risk of suicide are also characterized by pain syndromes. More than half of the patients with multiple sclerosis have pain that may not be recognized by treatment professionals. In this disorder, many patients report that pain is among the worst of their symptoms.

Pain is not always recognized as part of the symptoms of a chronic disorder. In such cases, complaints of pain may be neglected, and consequently the patient does not receive proper treatment of the pain.

Pain in addition to depression and feelings of hopelessness may enhance the patients choice of suicide as a solution to their problems.

Does the Patient Have a Crisis Reaction?

As demonstrated in Chapter 2, a crisis reaction occurs in the diagnostic period—a period with increased risk of suicide as seen in patients with cancer and neurological disorders.

How Is the Condition at Home?

Frequently, social consequences are a result of the disease. The patient's financial security changes. Retiring from work with financial problems, the patient may experience isolation as a consequence. Family and friends may withdraw from the patient. The result of all this may add to pain, depression, and a crisis reaction, thus increasing the risk of suicide.

When Was the Diagnosis Made?

In the prediagnostic period, uncertainty of the nature of the symptoms or genetic tests (Huntington's chorea) may precipitate suicide or suicide attempts.

The diagnostic period is a high-risk period for suicide, as has been seen in patients with cancer and neurological disorders. However, the postdiagnostic period can also be associated with risk of suicide, especially when the patient realizes the cost of living with a chronic disorder (renal dialysis, multiple sclerosis, diabetes mellitus) or when treatment promises do not fulfill the patients expectations (renal and liver transplants).

How Is Suicide Prevented?

When the clinician has realized that a risk of suicide exists, the next question is. How is the suicide prevented?

Acknowledge the Risk of Suicide

It is important to discuss the disease with the patient in order to get an impression of the patient's reaction to the disorder and the resources and network in the individual patient. Crisis reactions should be diagnosed and properly treated. Frequently, clinicians think that discussing suicidal thoughts may precipitate a suicide. However, usually the patient is relieved by being allowed to discuss his feelings and thoughts.

A need for psychiatric treatment of mental disorders such as depression may be revealed in the discussion with the patient. In some studies, diabetic patients were examined by a psychiatrist, but only one-third of the patients received the antidepressant treatment suggested by the psychiatrist (Lustman, Amado, and Wetzel, 1983; Lustman et al., 1983). Frequently, their depression was conceived as a natural and understandable reaction to a severe disease; thus, they did not receive treatment.

Antidepressant treatment has been tried in cancer patients, but the results were not impressive (Noyes and Kathal, 1986; Petty and Noyes, 1981; Rodin and Voshart, 1986). Better results have been found in patients with neurological disorders. However, an advantage in antidepressive drugs and neuroleptics is their pain-alleviating potential.

Finally, medication is not always the answer in reactive conditions. Discussions and counseling as well as explanations of symptoms, problems, and doubts should always be offered by competent clinicians. Medication may supplement this approach.

Treatment of Pain

Most pain can be reduced by sufficient pain treatment. Reducing pain will improve quality of life and reduce risk of suicide.

It is important to recognize and acknowledge the disorders associated with pain, and consequently treat them, perhaps by consulting experts on pain treatment.

Psychosocial Intervention

Chronic or life-threatening disease will affect both the patient and his or her relatives. Counseling on treatment, prognosis, and the social and human implications of the disease will usually be very helpful.

Furthermore, it is important that the clinician's responsibility for treatment does not stop when it becomes evident that a cure is not available for chronic, incapacitating disorders. Treatment responsibility also includes an obligation to secure the patient the best available quality of life in the time he or he has to live. Frequently, this will demand regular follow-ups in outpatient clinics, instead of leaving the postdiagnostic treatment entirely to the family physician. A practitioner will often face the problem of not knowing in detail all disorders, which makes it impossible to provide optimal care and counseling in the period immediately following diagnosis. In this period the patient will need regular controls in an expert outpatient clinic, which should be able to give adequate counseling.

In most places, psychosocial intervention requires a change in attitude toward patients with chronic disorders that have no available cures. Of course, national and regional differences exist on the possibilities of securing an optimal pychosocial treatment for these patients.

Periods with Risk of Suicide

As previously pointed out, the highest risk of suicide is in the diagnostic period, and the period immediately after the diagnosis. However, during genetic testing and in the postdiagnostic period, the risk still exists. Therefore, the clinician should always have the risk of suicide in mind.

Should Suicide Always Be Prevented?

Finally, we have to ask some controversial questions. Why is it important to prevent suicide? Should it not be the right of anyone to decide on a rational basis whether or not to commit suicide when suffering from an incurable disease?

The opposite question would be: When is the decision on suicide rationally based?

In studies on the frequency of mental disorders in cancer patients showed that 20 to 40 percent suffered from depression, and at an advanced stage of the disease, the figure was 77 percent (Noyes and Kathal, 1986; Petty and Noyes, 1981; Rodin and Vashart, 1986). More than half of the patients had conditions characterized by anxiety and depressed moods. A large portion of the patients had considerable pain. Whether or not such a condition is a rational basis for committing suicide is debatable.

Furthermore, studies on patients after a suicide attempt have demonstrated that very few made the attempt after careful consideration. Most frequently, it was an act of affect, released by a human problem. Thus, it was not a rational act.

Obviously, it is very difficult to decide whether or not the act is rational in patients who commit suicide. Psychological autopsy (Runeson, 1989; Stenager, Koch-Henriksen, and Stenager, 1996) and reviewing the available information are the only possibilities. Studies have shown that persons who commit suicide frequently had both mental and somatic disorders. Only a minority consulted medical and social services just prior to the suicide. Therefore, determining if all treatment options have been used is impossible.

Previous studies (Stenager and Jensen, 1994; Damsbo and Friborg, 1989; Diekstra and van Egmond, 1989) have shown that almost two-thirds of patients who attempt suicide have consulted the family physician or social services in a short time interval before the attempt. Stenager and Jensen (1994) demonstrated that patients with depression or pain more frequently consulted the physician before the attempt than other patients with suicide attempts. Frequently, the patients present other problems than suicidal thoughts. This may indicate that the suicidal behavior was not a rational act.

What Questions Should Be Asked of a Patient at Risk of Suicide?

The next part presents suggestions for questions that could be asked a patient expressing suicidal thoughts. The purpose of these questions is to evaluate the depth and rational basis of the expressed death wish.

- Is the patient asking for help?
- Why is the patient asking for help?
- What has kept the patient from suicide until now?
- Does the patient want someone else to take control?
- Is the suicidal wish stable and continuous?
- Is the wish coherent with the basic values of the patient?
- Is the medical information correct?
- Has the patient understood the information?
- Is the suicidal wish financially conditioned?
- Has the patient considered the reaction of family and others?
- Is the patient afraid of becoming a burden?
- Is the decision influenced by cultural conditions?
- Is the patient's support network functioning?
- Has the method been considered carefully?
- Is the patient going to tell others about the plans?
- Is suicide the only solution?
- Is the suicide rationally planned?

CONCLUSION

Patients with a number of chronic somatic disorders have an increased risk of suicide. The risk is highest in the period immediately after the diagnosis has been made, especially in patients with cancer and neurological disorders such as multiple sclerosis. Many reasons explain the increased risk.

Disorders resulting in an increased risk of suicide are also associated with an increased risk of mental disorders such as depression, anxiety disorders, and delirious conditions, which may be organically or medicamentously caused. Additionally, many patients will have a crisis reaction after diagnosis and during progression of the disease. They feel that their situation is hopeless. This feeling can increase depression as well as pain, a result that is frequent in both acute and chronic disorders.

It is important to understand which sufferings can be associated with a suicidal risk and be open to this possibility when counseling patients.

Furthermore, clinicians should also acknowledge the responsibility of treatment in patients with chronic, incapacitating, or life-threatening disorders after the possibility of a cure has vanished. Treatment also encompasses helping the patient obtain the best available quality of life in the remaining period he has to live. This demands continuous counseling and support. The treating physician has an enormous responsibility because he is the best person to explain the consequences of the disease to the patient. In some medical institutions, this responsibility is transferred to psychologists, nurses, social workers, and others who do not necessarily have as extensive knowledge of such issues as the treating physician does. This will influence the counseling negatively.

However, hospital staff is increasingly aware of these needs. Still, it is often felt that it is more convenient to take another blood test or radiological test than to sit down, listen, and talk with the patient.

Bibliography

Chapter 1

Åsberg M, Träskman L, Thoren P. (1976). 5-HIAA in cerebrospinal fluid: A biochemical suicide predictor? *Arch Gen Psychiatry* 33: 1193-1197.

Bille-Brahe U. (1993). WHO/EURO Multicentre on parasuicide. Facts and Figures. Copenhagen: World Health Organization. EUR/ICP/PSF 018.

Buzan RD, Weissberg MP. (1992). Suicide: Risk factors and prevention in medical practice. *Ann Rev Med* 43: 37-46.

Monk M. (1987). Epidemiology of suicide. *Epidimiologic Reviews* 9: 51-69.

Nielsen B. (1994). "Prædiktorer for gentagen suicidal adfærd." PhD thesis. Odense, Denmark: Odense University Press.

Nielsen B, Wang AG, Bille-Brahe U. (1990). Attempted suicide in Denmark IV: A five-year follow up. *Acta Psychiatr Scand* 81: 250-254.

Roy A, De Jong J, Linnoila M. (1989). Cerebrospinal fluid monoamine metabolites and suicidal behavior in depressed patient. A five-year follow-up study. *Arch Gen Psychiatry* 46: 609-612.

Stenager EN. (1996). "Attempted suicide: Treatment and outcome." PhD thesis. Odense, Denmark: Odense University Press.

Stenager EN, Benjaminsen S. (1991). Repetition of parasuicide, psychiatric diagnosis, and treatment modalities. A one-year follow up. In *Suicide attempts in the Nordic countries: Epidemiology and treatment*, T Bjerke, TC Stiles (eds.). Trondheim, Norway: Tapir Publishers, pp. 171-183.

Stenager EN, Jensen K. (1994). Attempted suicide: Contact to the primary health authorities. *Acta Psychiatrica Scand* 90: 109-113.

Träskman Bendz L, Alling C, Oreland L, Regnell G, Vinge E, Öhman R. (1992). Prediction of suicidal behaviour from biological tests. *J Clin Psychopharmacol* 12: 21S-26S.

WHO Regional Office for Europe. (1985). *Target for health for all: The health policy in Europe.* Copenhagen: WHO Regional Office for Europe (European Health for All Series. No.1).

Chapter 2

Brooks NA, Matson RR. (1982). Social-psychological adjustment to multiple sclerosis. A longitudinal study. *Soc Sci Med* 16: 2129-2135.

Büchi S, Buddeberg C, Sieber M. (1989). Die Bedeutung somatischer und psychosoziazialer Faktoren für die Krankheitsverarbeitung von Multiple-Sklerose-Kranken. *Der Nervenarzt* 60: 641-646.

Burnfield A. (1984). Doctor-patient dilemmas in multiple sclerosis. *J Med Ethics* 1: 24-26.

Burnfield A, Burnfield P. (1978). Common psychological problems in MS. *BMJ* 1: 1193-1194.

Burnfield A, Burnfield P. (1982). Psychosocial aspects of MS. *Physiother* 68: 149-150.

Catanzaro M, Weinert C. (1992). Economic status of families living with multiple sclerosis. *Int J Rehab Res* 15: 209-218.

Confavreux C, Aimard G, Devic M. (1980). Course and prognosis of multiple sclerosis assessed by computerized data processing of 349 patients. *Brain* 103: 281-300.

Duval ML. (1984). Psychosocial metaphors of physical distress among MS patients. *Soc Sci Med* 19: 635-638.

Elian M, Dean G. (1985). To tell or not to tell the diagnosis of MS. *Lancet* 6/7: 27-28.

Grønning M, Hannisdal E, Mellgren SI. (1990). Multivariate analysis of factors associated with unemployment in people with multiple sclerosis. *J Neurol Neurosurg Psychiatry* 53: 388-390.

Lauer K, Firnhaber W. (1987). Epidemiological investigations into multiple sclerosis in Southern Hesse. V Course and prognosis. *Acta Neurol Scand* 76: 12-17.

Marteux R. (1991). La Sclérose en plaques au quotidien. Santé, Paris: Editions Odile Jacob, p. 192.

Matson RR, Brooks NA. (1977). Adjusting to multiple sclerosis: An exploratory study. *Soc Sci Med* 11: 245-250.

Poser S, Kurtzke JF, Poser W, Schlaf G. (1989). Survival in multiple sclerosis. *Clin Epidemiol* 42: 159-168.

Spackman AJ, Roberts MHW, Martin JP, McLellan DL. (1989). Caring at night for people with multiple sclerosis. *BMJ* 299: 1433.

Spencer W. (1988). Suspicion of multiple sclerosis. To tell or not to tell? *Arch Neurol* 45: 441-442.

Stenager E, Jensen K. (1988). Multiple sclerosis: Correlation of psychiatric admissions to onset of initial symptoms. *Acta Neurol Scand* 77: 414-417.

Stenager E, Jensen K. (1993). Multiple sclerosis interpreted as surgical disease. *J Neurol Orthop Med Surg* 14: 19-22.

Stenager E, Knudsen L, Jensen K. (1989). When should the patient with multiple sclerosis be told his diagnosis? In *Mental disorders and cognitive deficits in multiple sclerosis*, K Jensen, L Knudsen, E Stenager, I Grant (eds.). London: John Libbey and Co. Ltd., pp. 191-195.

Stenager E, Knudsen L, Jensen K. (1991). Multiple sclerosis: The impact of physical impairment and cognitive dysfunction on social and spare time activities. *Psychother Psychosom* 56: 123-128.

Stenager E, Stenager EN, Knudsen L, Jensen K. (1994). Multiple sclerosis: The impact on family and social life. *Acta Psychiatrica Belg* 94: 165-174.

Stewart DC, Sullivans TJ. (1982). Illness and the sick role in chronic disease. *Soc Sci Med* 16: 1397-1404.

Thompson AJ, Kermode AG, MacManus DG, Kendall BE, Kingsley DPE, Moseley IF, McDonald WI. (1990). Patterns of disease activity in multiple sclerosis: Clinical and magnetic resonance study. *BMJ* 300: 631-634.
Weinshenker BG, Bass B, Rice GPA, Noseworthy J, Carriere W, Baskerville J, Ebers GC. (1989). The natural history of multiple sclerosis: A geographically based study. I Clinical course and disability. *Brain* 112: 133-146.

Chapter 3

Allgulander C. (1994). Suicide and mortality patterns in anxiety neurosis and depressive neurosis. *Arch Gen Psychiatry* 52: 708-712.
Allgulander C, Fisher LD. (1990). Clinical predictors of completed suicide and repeated self-poisoning in 8,895 self-poisoning patients. *Eur Arch Psychiatry Neurol Sci* 239: 270-276.
Arato'M, Demeter E, Rihmer Z, Somogyi E. (1988). Retrospective psychiatric assessment of 200 suicides in Budapest. *Acta Psychiatrica Scand* 77: 454-456.
Åsgård U. (1990). A psychiatric study of suicide among urban Swedish women. *Acta Psychiatrica Scand* 82: 115-124.
Babigian HM, Odoroff CL. (1969). The mortality experience of a population with psychiatric illness. *Am J Psychiatry* 126: 470-480.
Barner-Rasmussen P, Dupont A, Bille H. (1986). Suicide in psychiatric patients in Denmark, 1971-81. I. Demographic and diagnostic description. *Acta Psychiatry Scand* 73: 441-448.
Barraclough B, Bunch J, Nelson B, Sainsbury P. (1974). A hundred cases of suicide: Clinical aspects. *Brit J Psychiatry* 125: 355-373.
Beskow J. (1979). Suicide and mental disorders in Swedish men 1970-1971. *Acta Pychiatrica Scand* (suppl 277).
Black DW, Warrack G, Winokur G. (1985). Excess mortality among psychiatric patients. *JAMA* 253: 58-61.
Bleuler M. (1978). The schizophrenic disorders: Long-term family studies. New Haven, CT: Yale University Press.
Brown T, Sheran T. (1972). Suicide prediction: A review. *Life-Threatening Behaviour* 2: 67-98.
Chynoweth R, Tonnge JL, Amstrong J. (1980). Suicide in Brisbane: A retrospective psychosocial study. *Aust N Z J Psychiatry* 14: 37-45.
Coryell W. (1988). Panic disorder and mortality. *Psychiatric clinics of North America* 11(2): 433-440.
Dorpat TL, Ripley HS. (1960). A study of suicide in the Seattle area. *Compr Psychiatry* 1: 349-359.
Dorpat TL, Ripley HS. (1967). The relationship between attempted suicide and committed suicide. *Compr Psychiatry* 8: 74-79.
Drake RE, Gates C, Whitaker A, Cotton PG. (1985). Suicide among schizophrenics: A review. *Compr Psychiatry* 26: 90-100.
Egmond van M, Diekstra RFW. (1990). The predictability of suicidal behavior: The results of a meta-analysis of published studies. *Crisis* 2: 57-84.

Ennis J, Barnes AB, Kennedy S, Trachtenberg DD. (1989). Depression in self-harm patients. *Br J Psychiatry* 54: 41-47.

Frances R, Franklin J, Flavin D. (1987). Suicide and alcoholism. *Am-J-Drug-Alcohol-Abuse* 13(3): 327-341.

Friedman S, Jones JC, Chernen L, Barlow DH. (1992). Suicidal ideation and suicide attempts among patients with panic disorder: A survey of two outpatient clinics. *Am J Psychiatry* 149: 680-685.

Guze SB, Robins E. (1970). Suicide and primary affective disorders. *Brit J Psychiatry* 117: 437-438.

Hagnell O, Lanke J, Rorsman B. (1981). Suicide rates in the Lundby study: Mental illness as a risk factor for suicide. *Neuropsychobiol* 7: 248-253.

Hagnell O, Rorsman B. (1987). Suicide and endogenous depression with somatic symptoms in the Lundby study. *Neuropsychobiol* 4: 180-187.

Hawton K, Fagg J. (1988). Suicide, and other causes of death following attempted suicide. *Brit J Psychiatry* 152: 359-366.

Isometsa ET, Henrikson MM, Aro HM, Lönnqvist JK. (1993). Mental disorders and comorbidity in suicide. *Am J Psychiatry* 150: 935-940.

Johnson J, Weissman MM, Klerman GL. (1990). Panic disorder, comorbidity, and suicide attempts. *Arch Gen Psychiatry* 47: 805-808.

Lester D. (1972). Why people kill themselves. Springfield, IL: Charles C Thomas.

Maris RW. (1981). *Pathway to suicide: A survey of self-destructive behaviour.* Baltimore: The Johns Hopkins University Press.

Miles C. (1977). Conditions predisposing to suicide: A review. *J Nerve Ment Dis* 164: 231-246.

Monk M. (1987). Epidemiology of suicide. *Epidemiologic Reviews* 9: 51-89.

Mortensen PB, Juel K. (1990). Mortality and causes of death in schizophrenic patients in Denmark. *Acta Psychiatrica Scand* 82: 372-2.

Murphy GE. (1986). Suicide in alcoholism. In *Suicide*, A Roy (ed.). Baltimore: Williams and Wilkins.

Murphy G, Wetzel R. (1990). The lifetime risk of suicide in alcoholism. *Arch Gen Psychiatry* 47: 383-392.

Nielsen B. "Prædiktorer for gentagen suicidal adfærd." (1994). PhD thesis. Odense, Denmark: Odense University Press.

Nielsen B, Wang AG, Bille-Brahe U. (1990). Attempted suicide in Denmark. IV. A five-year follow-up. *Acta Psychiatrica Scand* 81: 250-254.

Pitts FN Jr, Winokur G. (1966). Affective disorder. VII. Alcoholism and affective disorders. *J Psychiatry Res* 4: 37-50.

Pokorny AD. (1983). Prediction of suicide in psychiatric patients. *Arch Gen Psychiatry* 40: 249-257.

Rich CL, Young D, Fowler RC. (1986). The San Diego suicide study: I. Young vs. old subjects. *Arch Gen Psychiatry* 43: 577-582.

Robins E, Murphy GE, Wilkinson RH, Gassner S, Kayes J. (1959). Some clinical considerations in the prevention of suicide based on a study of 134 successful suicides. *Am J Public Health* 49: 888-899.

Roy A (ed.) (1986). *Suicide.* Baltimore: Williams and Wilkins.

Runeson B. (1989). Mental disorder in youth suicides. *Acta Psychiatry Scand* 79: 490-497.

Rygnestad T. (1988). A prospective five-year follow-up study of self-poisoned patients. *Acta Psychiatrica Scand* 77: 328-331.

Sainsbury P. (1986). Depression, suicide and suicide prevention. In *Suicide,* A Roy (ed.). Baltimore: Williams and Wilkins, pp. 73-88.

Stenager E. (1996). "Attempted suicide: Outcome and treatment." PhD thesis. Odense, Denmark: Odense University Press.

Stenager E, Christensen LL, Jepsen I, Krarup G, Pedersen P, Thygesen-Rasmussen G, Benjaminsen S. (1991). Selvmordsforsøg og depression. *Ugeskr Læger* 153: 836-839.

Stenager EN, Koch-Henriksen N, Stenager E. (1996). Risk factors for suicide in multiple sclerosis. *Psychother Psychosom* 65: 86-90.

Stenager EN, Christensen LL, Jepsen I, Krarup G, Pedersen P, Thygesen-Rasmussen G, Benjaminsen S. (1990). Depression in attempted suicide. In: *3rd European symposium: Suicidal behaviour and risk factors,* G Ferrari, M Belline, P Crepet (eds.). Bologna, Italy: Monduzzi, pp. 603-608.

Suokas J, Lønnquist J. (1991). Outcome of attempted suicide and psychiatric consultation. Risk factors and suicide mortality during a five-year follow-up. *Acta Psychiatrica Scand* 84: 545-549.

Tsuang MT. (1978). Suicide in schizophrenics, manics, depressives, and surgical controls. *Arch Gen Psychiatry* 35: 153-154.

Urwin P, Gibbons JL. (1979). Psychiatric diagnosis in self-poisoning patients. *Psychol Med* 9: 501-507.

Chapter 4

Allgulander C, Fisher LD. (1990). Clinical predictors of completed suicide and repeated self-poisoning in 8,895 self-poisoning patients. *Eur Arch Psychiatry Neurol Sci* 239: 2.

Barraclough BM. (1987). The suicide rate of epilepsy. *Acta Psychiatrica Scand* 76: 339-345.

Fishbain DA, Goldberg M, Rosomoff RS, Rosomoff H. (1991). Case report. Completed suicide in chronic pain. *Clin J Pain* 7: 29-36.

Guze SB, Robins E. (1970). Suicide among primary affective disorders. *Br J Psychiatry* 117: 437-438.

Mortensen PB, Juel K. (1990). Mortality and causes of death in schizophrenic patients in DK. *Acta Psychiatrica Scand* 81: 372-377.

Stenager EN, Stenager E. (1992). Suicide and patients with neurological diseases: Methodologic problems. *Arch Neurol* 49 : 1296-1303.

Stenager EN, Bille-Brahe U, Jensen K. (1991). Kræft og selvmord: En litteraturoversigt. *Ugeskr Læger* 153: 764-769.

Stenager E, Knudsen L, Jensen K. (1990). Psychiatric and cognitive aspects of multiple sclerosis. *Sem Neurol* 10(3): 254-261.

Stenager EN, Stenager E, Koch-Henriksen N, Brønnum-Hansen H, Hyllested K, Jensen K, Bille-Brahe U. (1992). Suicide in multiple sclerosis: An epidemiological study. *J Neurol Neurosurg Psychiatry* 55(7): 542-545.

Stensman R, Sundqvist-Stensman UB. (1988). Physical disease and disability among 416 cases in Sweden. *Scand J Soc Med* 16: 149-153.

Whitlock FA. (1982). The neurology of affective disorder and suicide. *Aust N Z J Psych* 16: 1-12.

Whitlock FA. (1985). Suicide and physical illness. In *Suicide*, A Roy (ed.). Baltimore: Williams and Wilkins, pp. 151-170.

Chapter 5

Achté KA, Lönnquist J, Hillbom E. (1971). Suicides following war brain-injuries. *Acta Psychiatrica Scand* (suppl 225): 3-92.

Allgulander C, Fisher LD. (1990). Clinical predictors of completed suicide and repeated self-poisoning in 8,895 self-poisoning patients. *Eur Arch Psychiatry Neurol Sci* 239: 270-276.

Bak S, Stenager EN, Stenager E, Boldsen J, Smith TA. (1994). Suicide in patients with motor neuron disease. *Behavioral Neurol* 7: 181-184.

Barraclough BM. (1987). The suicide rate of epilepsy. *Acta Psychiatrica Scand* 76: 339-345.

Charlifue SW, Gerhart KA. (1991). Behavioral and demographic predictors of suicide after traumatic spinal cord injury. *Arch Phys Med Rehab* 72: 488-492.

Chiu E, Aleksander L. (1982). Causes of death in Huntington's disease. *Med J Australia* 1: 153.

Cummings JL. (1992). Depression and Parkinson's disease: A review. *Am J Psychiatry* 149: 44-454.

DeVivo MS, Black KS, Scott Richards J, Stover SL. (1991). Suicide following spinal cord injury. *Paraplegia* 29: 620-627.

Farrer LA. (1986). Suicide and attempted suicide in Huntington's disease: Implications for preclinical testing of persons at risk. *Am J Med Gen* 24: 305-311.

Feigin G. (1988). Suicide and meningioma. *Am J for Med Path* 9: 334-335.

Folstein MF, Maiberger R, McHugh PR. (1977). Mood disorder as a specific complication of stroke. *J Neurol Neurosurg Psychiatry* 40: 1018-1020.

Frisbie JH, Kache A. (1983). Increasing survival and changing causes of death in myelopathy patients. *J Am Paraplegia Society* 6(3): 51-56.

Garden FH, Garrison SJ, Jain A. (1990). Assessing suicide risk in stroke patients: Review of two cases. *Arch Phys Med Rehab* 71: 1003-1005.

Geisler WO, Jousse AT, Wynne-Jones M. (1977). Survival in traumatic transverse myelitis. *Paraplegia* 14: 262-275.

Geisler WO, Jousse AT, Wynne-Jones M, Breithaupt D. (1983). Survival in traumatic spinal cord injury. *Paraplegia* 21: 364-373.

Henriksen PB, Juul-Jensen P, Lund M. (1970). The mortality of epileptics. Internat congress of life assurance medicine: Life assurance medicine. In RBC Brackenridge (ed.). London: Pittman, pp. 139-148.

Henry GW. (1932). Mental phenomena observed in cases of brain tumor. *Am J Psychiatry* 12: 415-473.

Hoehn MM, Yahr MD. (1967). Parkinsonism: Onset, progression and mortality. *Neurol* 17: 427-442.

Huntington G. (1872). On chorea: Medical and surgical reporter. 26: 317-321.

Ivanainen M, Lehtimen J. (1979). Causes of death in institutionalized epileptics. *Epilepsy* 30: 485-492.

Jackson JA, Free GBM, Pike HV. (1923). The psychic manifestations in paralysis agitans. *Arch Neurol Psychiatry* 10: 680-684.

Keschner M, Bender MB, Strauss I. (1938). Mental symptoms associated with brain tumor. *JAMA* 110: 714-718.

Kessler S. (1987). Psychiatric implications of presymptomatic testing for Huntington's disease. *Am J Orthopsychiatry* 57(2): 212-219.

Kurtzke JF, Beebe GW, Nagler W, Netzger MD, Auth TL, Kurland LT. (1970). Studies on the natural history of multiple sclerosis: Long-term survival in young men. *Arch Neurol* 22: 215-225.

Le CT, Price M. (1982). Survival from spinal cord injury. *J Chron Dis* 35: 487-492.

Leibowitz U, Kahana E, Alter M. (1971). Cerebral multiple sclerosis. *Neurol* 21: 1179-1185.

Lewin W, Marshall TFDeC, Roberts AH. (1979). Long-term outcome after severe head injury. *Brit Med J* 2: 1533-1538.

Matthews WS, Barabas G. (1981). Suicide and epilepsy: A review of the literature. *Psychosom* 22: 515-524.

Mayeux R, Williams JBW, Stern Y, Côte L. (1984). Depression and Parkinson's disease. *Adv Neurol* 40: 241-250.

McAlpine D, Lumsden CE, Acheson ED. (1972). *Multiple sclerosis: A reappraisal*, second edition. Baltimore: Williams and Wilkins Company.

Mindham RHS. (1970). Psychiatric symptoms in Parkinsonism. *J Neurol Neurosurg Psychiatry* 33: 188-191.

Müller R. (1949). Studies on disseminated sclerosis with special reference to symptomatology course and prognosis. *Acta Med Scand* 133(122).

Nyquist RH, Bors E. (1967). Mortality and survival in traumatic myelopathy during nineteen years from 1946 to 1965. *Paraplegia* 5: 22-47.

Oyebode F, Kennedy S, Davidson K. (August 1986). Psychiatric sequelae of subarachnoid hemorrhage. *Br J Hosp Med*: 104-108.

Parkinson J. (1817). *An essay on the shaking palsy*. London: Sherwood, Neely, and Jones.

Prudhomme C. (1941). Epilepsy and suicide. *J Nerv Ment Dis* 94: 722-731.

Reed TE, Chandler JH. (1958). Huntington's chorea in Michigan. *Am J Hum Genet* 10: 201-225.

Sadovnick AB, Ebers GC, Paty DW, Eisen K. (1985). Causes of death in multiple sclerosis. *Can J Neurol Sci* 12: 189.

Saugstad L, Ødegård Ø. (1979). Mortality in psychiatric hospitals in Norway 1950-74. *Acta Psychiatrica Scand* 59: 431-447.

Saugstad L, Ødegård Ø. (1986). Huntington's chorea in Norway. *Psychol Med* 16: 39-48.

Schneider E, Fischer PA, Jacobi P, Kolb R. (1981). Mortalität beim Parkinson-syndrom und ihre Beeinflussung durch L-Dopa. Fortschr. *Neurol Psychiat* 41: 187-192.

Schoenfeld M, Myers RH, Cupples LA, Berkman B, Sax Ds, Clark E. (1984). Increased rate of suicide among patients with Huntington's disease. *J Neurol Neurosurg Psychiatry* 47: 1283-1287.

Schwartz ML, Pierron M. (1972). Suicide and fatal accidents in multiple sclerosis. *Omega* 3: 291-293.

Stenager EN, Jensen K, Bille-Brahe U. (1991). Suicide and cancer: A review of the literature. *Ugeskr Læger* 11: 764-768.

Stenager EN, Stenager E, Jensen K. (1991). Suizid bei Patienten mit Multipler Sclerose. In *Krankheit und Suizid*, H Wedler, HJ Müller (eds.). Regensburg, Germany: Roderer Verlag.

Stenager EN, Wermuth L, Stenager E, Boldsen J. (1994). Suicide in patients with Parkinson's disease. *Acta Psychiatry Scand* 90: 70-72.

Stenager EN, Stenager E, Koch-Henriksen N, Brønnum-Hansen H, Hyllested K, Jensen K, Bille-Brahe U. (1992). Multiple sclerosis and suicide: An epidemiological study. *J Neurol Neurosurg and Psychiatry* 55: 542-545.

Stensman R, Sundqvist-Stensman UB. (1988). Physical disease and disability among 416 cases on Schweden. *Scand J Soc Med* 16: 149-153.

Vaukonen K. (1959). Suicide among the male with war injuries to the brain. *Acta Psychiatrica et Neurol Scand* 137: 90-91.

Wermuth L, Stenager EN, Stenager E, Boldsen J. (1995). Mortality in patients with Parkinson's disease. *Acta Neurol Scand* 92: 55-58.

White SJ, McLean AEM, Howland C. (1979). Anticonvulsant drugs and cancer. *Lancet* 2: 458-461.

Whitlock FA. (1982). The neurology of affective disorder and suicide. *Aust N Z J Psych* 16: 1-12.

Whitlock FA. (1986). Suicide and physical illness. In *Suicide*, A Roy (ed.). Baltimore: Williams and Wilkins, pp. 151-170.

Zielenski JJ. (1974). Mortality and cause of death of epileptics. *Epilepsy* 15: 191-201.

Chapter 6

Allebeck P, Bolund C, Ringbäck G. (1989). Increased suicide rate in cancer patients. *J Clin Epidemiol* 42(7): 611-616.

Beck AT, Steer RA, Kovacs M, Garrison B. (1985). Hopelessness and eventual suicide: A 10-year prospective study of patients hospitalized with suicidal ideation. *Am J Psychiatry* 5: 559-563.

Bolund C. (1985). Suicide and cancer: I. Demographic and social characteristics of cancer patients who committed suicide in Schweden, 1973-1976. *J Psychosocial Oncol* 3(1): 17-30.

Bolund C. (1985). Suicide and cancer: II. Medical and care factors in suicides by patients in Schweden, 1973-1976. *J Phychosocial Oncol* 3(1): 31-52.

Campbell PC. (1966). Suicide among cancer patients. *Health Bull* 80(9): 207-212.

Dorpat TL, Ripley HS. (1960). A study of suicide in the Seattle area. *Compr Psychiatry* 1: 349-359.

Derogatis LR, Morrow GR, Fetting J, Penman D, Piasetsky S, Schmale AM, Henrichs M, Carnicke CLM. (1983). The prevalence of psychiatric disorders among cancer patients. *JAMA* 249(6): 751-757.

Farberow N, Ganzler S, Cutter F, Reynolds D. (1971). An eight-year survey of hospital suicides. *Suicide and Life-Threatening Behav* 1(3): 184-202.

Fox BH, Stanek EJ, Boyd SC, Flannery JT. (1982). Suicide rates among cancer patients in Connecticut. *J Chron Dis* 35: 89-100.

Gezelius C, Eriksson A. (1988). Neoplastic disease in a medicolegal autopsy materal: A retrospective study in Northern Sweden. *Z Rechtsmedizin* 101: 115-130.

Hjortsjö T. (1987). Suicide in relation to somatic illness and complications. *Crisis* 8(2): 125-137.

Levi F, Builliard JL, La Vecchia C. (1991). Suicide risk among incident cases of cancer in the Swiss canton Vaud. *Oncol* 48: 44-47.

Louhivouri KA, Hakama M. (1979). Risk of suicide among cancer patients. *Am J Epidemiol* 109(1): 59-64.

Lynch ME. (1995). The assessment and prevalence of affective disorders in advanced cancer. *J Palliative Care* 1: 1-18.

Marshall JR, Burnett W, Brasure J. (1983). On precipitating factors: Cancer as a cause of suicide. *Suicide and Life-Threatening Behav* 13(1): 15-27.

Murphy GK. (1977). Cancer and the coroner. *JAMA* 8: 786-788.

Olafsen OM. (1981). Suicide among cancer patients in Norway. In *Depression et crime*, JP Soubrier, J Wedrinne (eds.). New York: Pergamon Press, pp. 587-591.

Noyes R. Kathol RG. (1986). Depression and cancer. *Psychiatric Developments* 2: 77-100.

Perrone. (1993). Adolescents with cancer: Are they at risk for suicide? *Pediatric Nursing* 19: 22-25.

Pollak S, Missliwetz J. (1979). Selbsttötungen in Wiener Krankenhäusern. *Z Rechtsmedizin* 233-244.

Plumb M, Holland J. (1981). Comparative studies of psychological function in patients with advanced cancer II. Interviewer-rated current and past psychological symptoms. *Psychomatic Med* 43(3): 243-254.

Petty F, Noyes R. (1981). Depression secondary to cancer. *Biological Psychiatry* 16(12): 1203-1220.

Richards SH. (1994). Finding the means to carry on. Suicidal feelings in cancer patients. *Professional Nurse* 9: 334-339.

Rodin G, Voshart K. (1986). Depression in the medically ill: An overview. *J Psychiatry* 143(6): 696-705.

Sainsbury P. (1955). *Suicide in London*. London: Chapman and Hall, 8-83.

————. (1986). Depression, suicide, and suicide prevention. In *Suicide*, A Roy (ed.). Baltimore: Williams and Wilkins, pp. 73-88.

Saunders JM, Valente SM. (1988). Cancer and suicide. *Oncology Nursing Forum* 5: 575-581.

Stenager EN, Jensen K, Bille-Brahe U. (1991). Suicide and cancer: A review. *Ugeskr Læger* 153: 764-769.

Stenager EN, Stenager E, Jensen K. (1992). Selbstmord bei Patienten mit Multipler Sklerose. In *Krankheit und Suizid*, H Wedler, HJ Müller (eds.). Regensburg, Germany: Roderer Verlag, pp. 869-872.

Stensman R, Sundqvist-Stensman UB. (1988). Physical disease and disability among 416 suicide cases in Sweden. *Scand J Soc Med* 16: 149-153.

Stiefel F, Volkenaandt M, Breitbart W. (1989). Suicide and cancer. *Schweiz Med Wochenschr* 119(25): 891-895.

Storm HH, Christensen C, Jensen OM. (1992). Suicide, violent death, and cancer. *Cancer* 69: 1507-1512.

Whitlock FA. (1978). Suicide, cancer, and depression. *Brit J Psychiatry* 132: 269-274.

Whitlock FA. (1986). Suicide and physical illness. In *Suicide*, A Roy (ed.). Baltimore: Williams and Wilkins, pp. 151-170.

Chapter 7

Abram HS, Moore G, Vestervelt FB. (1971). Suicidal behaviour in chronic dialysis patients. *Am J Psychiatry* 127: 1199-1204.

Åsberg M, Nordstrøm P, Träskman-Bendz L. (1986). Biological factors in suicide. In *Suicide*, A Roy (ed.). London: Williams and Wilkins, pp. 47-71.

Åsberg M, Traskman L, Thoren P. (1976). 5-HIAA in cerebrospinal fluid: A biochemical suicide predictor. *Arch Gen Psychiatry* 33: 1193-1197.

Bakalim G. (1969). Causes of death in a series of 4,738 Finnish war amputees. *Artificial Limbs* 13: 27-36.

Berglund M. (1986). Suicide in male alcoholics with peptic ulcers. *Alcoholism* 10: 631-634.

Bonnevie O. (1977). Causes of death in duodenal and gastric ulcer. *Gastroenterol* 73: 1000-1004.

Burton HJ, Kline SA, Lindsay RM, Heidenheim AP. (1986). The relationship of depression to survival in chronic renal failure. *Psychosom Med* 48: 261-269.

Conwell Y. (1995). Nutrition. *Crisis* 16: 56-58.

Cooke WT, Mallas E, Prior P, Allan RN. (1980). Crohn's disease: Course, treatment, and long-term prognosis. *Quarterly J Med* 49: 363-384.

Coté TR, Biggar RJ, Dannenberg AL (1992). Risk of suicide among persons with AIDS: A national assessment. *JAMA* 268: 2066-2068.

Deckert T, Poulsen JE, Larsen M. (1978). Prognosis of diabetics with diabetes onset before the age of thirtyone. *Diabetologia* 14: 363-370.

Dorpat TL, Ripley HS. (1960). A study of suicide in the Seattle area. *Compr Psychiatry* 1: 349-359.

Drummond L, Lodrick M, Hallstrom C. (1984). Thyroid abnormalities and violent suicide. *Br J Psychiatry* 144: 213.

Erlandson SI, Archer T. (1994). Tinnitus, pain, and affective disorders. In *Strategies for studying brain disorders, volume 1: Depressive, anxiety and drug abuse disorders*, T Palomo, T Archer (eds.). London: Farrand Press.

Farberow NL, Ganzler S, Cutter E, Reynolds D. (1971). An 8-year survey of hospital suicides. *Suicide and Life-Threatening Behav* 1: 184-202.

Farberow NL, McKelligott JW, Cohen S, Darbonne A. (1966). Suicide among patients with cardiorespiratory illnesses. *JAMA* 195: 128-134.

Goodkin G. (1975). Mortality factors in diabetes: A 20-year mortality study. *J. Occupational Med* 17: 716-721.

Grüner OPN, Naas R, Gjone E, Flatmark A, Fretheim B. (1987). Mental disorders in ulcerative colitis: Suicide, divorce, hospitalization for mental disease, alcoholism, and consumption of psychotropic drugs in 178 patients subjected to colectomi. *Diseases of the Colon and Rectum* 21: 37-39.

Haenel Th, Brunner F, Battegay R. (1980). Renal dialysis and suicide: Occurrence in Switzerland and in Europe. *Compr Psychiatry* 21: 140-145.

Hagnell O, Wretmark G. (1957). Peptic ulcer and alcoholism: A statistical study in frequency, behavior, personality traits, and family occurrence. *J Psychosom Res* 2: 35-44.

Harrop-Griffith J, Katon W, Bobie R, Sakai C, Russo J. (1987). Chronic tinnitus: Association with psychiatric diagnosis. *J Psychosom Res* 31: 613-621.

Haskett RF. (1985). Diagnostic categorization of psychiatric disturbance in Cushing's syndrome. *Am J Psychiatry* 142: 911-916.

Hjortsjö T. (1987). Suicide in relation to somatic illness and complications. *Crisis* 8(2): 125-137.

Hrubec Zdenek, Ryder RA. (1979). Report to the Veteran's Administration Department of Medicine and Surgery on service connected traumatic limb amputations and subsequent mortality from cardiovascular disease and other causes of death. *Bull Prosthetics Res* 16: 29-53.

Jacobs D, Blackburn H, Higgins M, Reed D, Iso H, Mcmillan G, Neaton J, Nelson J, Potter J, Rifkind B, Rossouw J, Shekelle R, Yusuf S. (1992). Report of the conference on low blood cholesterol mortality associations. *Circulation* 86: 1046-1060.

Joner G, Patrick S. (1991). The mortality of children with type 1 (insulin-dependent) diabetes mellitus in Norway, 1973-1988. *Diabetologia* 34: 29-32.

Kizer KW, Green M, Perkins CI, Doebbert G, Hughes MJ. (1988). AIDS and suicide in California. *JAMA* 260: 1881.

Knop J, Fischer A. (1981). Duodenal ulcer, suicide, psychopathology, and alcoholism. *Acta Psychiatrica Scand* 63: 346-355.

Krause U. (1963). Long-term results of medical and surgical treatment of peptic ulcer. *Acta Chirurgica Scandinavia* 310 (suppl).

Kyvik K, Stenager E, Green A, Svendsen A. (1994). Suicides in men with IDDM. *Diabetes Care* 17: 210-212.

LaRosa JC. (1995). Cholesterol lowering and morbidity and mortality. *Current Opinion in Lipidol* 6: 62-65.

Lewis JE, Stephens SDG, McKenna L. (1994). Tinnitus and suicide. *Clin Otolaryngeol* 19: 50-54.

Linkowski P, vanWettere JP, Kerkhofs M, Brauman H, Medlewicz J. (1983). Thyrotrophin response to thyreostimulin in affectively ill woman: Relationship to suicidal behavior. *Brit J Psychiatry* 143: 401-405.

Lustman PJ, Amado H, Wetzel RD. (1983). Depression in diabetics: A critical appraisal. *Compr Psychiatry* 24(1): 65-74.

Lustman PJ, Griffith LS, Clouse RE, Cryer PE. (1986). Psychiatric illness in diabetes mellitus relationship to symptoms and glucose control. *J Nervous and Mental Dis* 174(12): 736-742.

MacGregor M. (1977). Juvenile diabetics growing up. *Lancet* 1: 944-945.

Marks HH, Krall LP. (1971). Onset, course, prognosis, and morbidity in diabetes mellitus. In *Joslins Diabetes Mellitus*, A Marble, P White, RF Bradley, LP Krall (eds.). Philadelphia: Lea and Febiger, p. 11.

Marzuk PM, Tierney H, Tardiff K, Gross EM, Morgan EB, Ming-An HSU, Mann JJ. (1988). Increased suicide risk of suicide in persons with AIDS. *JAMA* 259: 1333-1337.

Montandon A, Frey FJ. (1991). Decreased risk of suicide in renal transplant patients on cyclosporin. *Lancet* 338: 635.

Neaton JD, Blackburn H, Jacobs D, Kuller L, Lee DJ, Sherwin R, Shih J, Stamler J, Wentworth D. (1992). Serum cholesterol level and mortality findings for men screened in the Multiple Risk Factor Intervention Trial. *Arch Int Medicine* 152: 1490-1500.

North CS, Ray EC, Spitznael EL, Alpers DH. (1990). The relation of ulcerative colitis to psychiatric factors: A review of findings and methods. *Am J Psychiatry* 147: 974-981.

Perry S, Jacobsberg L, Fishman B. (1990). Suicidal ideation and HIV testing. *JAMA* 263: 679-682.

Pollak S, Missliwetz J. (1979). Selbsttötungen in Wiener Krankenhäusern. *Z Rechtsmedizin* 83(3): 233-244.

Popkin MK, Callies AL, Lentz RD, Colon EA, Sutherland DE. (1988). Prevalence of major depression, simple phobia, and other psychiatric disorders in patients with long-standing Type I diabetes mellitus. *Arch Gen Psychiatry* 45: 64-68.

Radford EP, Doll R, Smith PG. (1977). Mortality among patients with ankylosing spondylitis not given X-ray therapy. *NEJM* 297: 572-576.

Riether AM, Mahler E. (1994). Suicide in liver transplant patients. *Psychosom* 35: 574-577.

Robinson N, Fuller JH, Edmeades SP. (1988). Depression and diabetes. *Diabetic Med* 5: 168-174.

Ross AHAM, Smith MA, Anderson JR, Small WP. (1982). Late mortality after surgery for peptic ulcer. *NEJM* 307: 519-522.

Sainsbury P. (1955). *Suicide in London*. London: Chapman and Hall, 81-83.

Sawyer JD, Adams KM, Conway WL, Reeves J, Kvale PA. (1983). Suicide in cases of chronic obstructive pulmonary disease. *J Psychiatr Treatment and Evaluation* 5: 281-283.

Shapiro S, Waltzer H. (1980). Successful suicides and serious attempts in a general hospital over a 15 year period. *Gen Hosp Psychiatry* 2: 118-126.

Sheffield BF, Garney MWP. (1976). Crohn's disease: A psychosomatic illness. *Brit J Psychiatry* 128: 446-450.

Shukla GD, Sahu SC, Tripathi RP, Gupta DK. (1982). A psychiatric study of amputees. *Brit J Psychiatry* 141: 50-53.

Starr AM. (1952). Personality changes in Cushing's syndrome. *J Clin Endocrinol and Metab* 12: 502-505.

Stensman R, Sundqvist-Stensman UB. (1988). Physical disease and disability among 416 suicide cases in Sweden. *Scand J Soc Med* 16: 149-153.

Stewart I, Leeds MD. (1960). Suicide: The influence of organic diseases. *Lancet*: 919-920.

Taft P, Martin FIR, Melick R. (1970). Cushing's syndrome: A review of the response to treatment in 42 patients. *Aust Ann Med* 4: 295-303.

Tuckman J, Youngman WF, Keizman G. (1966). Suicide an physical illness. *J G Psychol* 75: 291-295.

Tunbridge WMG. (1981). Factors contributing to deaths of diabetics under fifty years of age. *Lancet* 2: 569-572.

Viskum K. (1975). Ulcer, attempted suicide, and suicide. *Acta Psychiatry Scand* 51: 221-227.

Washer GF, Schröter GPJ, Starzl TE, Weill R. (1983). Causes of death after kidney transplantation. *JAMA* 250: 49-54.

Wedler H. (1991). Körperliche Krankheiten bei Suizidpatienten einer internistischen Abteilung. In *Körperliche Krankheit und Suizid*, H Wedler, HJ Möller (eds.). Regensburg, Germany: Roderer S Verlag, pp. 87-101.

Wells KB, Golding JM, Burnam MA. (1988). Pychiatric disorders in a sample of the general population with and without chronic medical conditions. *Am J Psychiatry* 145: 976-981.

Wells KB, Golding JM, Burnam MA. (1989). Affective, substance use, and anxiety disorders in persons with arthritis, diabetes, heart disease, high blood pressure, or chronic lung condition. *Gen Hosp Psychiatry* 11: 320-327.

Westlund K. (1963). Mortality of peptic ulcer patient's. *Acta Med Scand* (suppl 402).

Westlund K. (1969). Mortality of diabetics. Oslo, Universitetsforlaget: Norwegian Monographs on Medical Science.

Whitlock FA. (1986). Suicide and physical illness. In *Suicide*, A Roy (ed.). Baltimore: Williams and Wilkins, pp. 151-170.

Wolfersdorf VM. (1988). Depression und suizid bei körperlichen Krankheiten. *Fortschritt Med* 106: 269-274.

Chapter 8

Arem R, Zogbi W. (1985). Insulin overdose in eight patients: Insulin pharmacokinetics and review of the literature. *Medicine* 64(5): 323-332.

Åsberg M, Nordstrøm P, Träskman-Bendz L. (1986). Biological factors in suicide, In *Suicide*, A Roy (ed.). Baltimore: Williams and Wilkins, pp. 47-73.

Bille-Brahe U. (1993). Background documents of the WHO/EURO Multicentre Study on Parasuicide. Document EUR/ICO/PSF 018).

Bourgeois M. (1974). Suicides insuliniques un nouveau cas d'injections massives d'insuline chez une diabétique. *Societe Medico-Psychologique*: 631-640.

Bourgeois M, Dufourg J. (1967). Suicides insuliniques. *Societe Medico-Psychologique*: 133-140.

Breslau N, Davis GC, Andreski P. (1991). Migraine, psychiatric disorders, and suicide attempts: An epidemiological study of young adults. *Psychiatry Research* 37: 11-23. 14.

Chalier M. (1969). Suicides et tentatives de suicide par l'insuline a propos de 39 observations dont une originale. *These de medecine* (Lyon) 107.

Dietzfelbinger T, Kurz A, Torhorst A, Möller HJ. (1991). Körperliche ind seelishe Krankheit als Hintergrund parsuizidalens Verhaltens. In *Körperliche Krankheit und Suizid*, H Wedler, HJ Möller (eds.). Regensburg, Germany: Roderer S Verlag, pp. 101-115.

Dubovsky SL. (1978). Averting suicide in terminally ill patients. *Psychomatics* 19(2): 113-115.

Gale E. (1980). Hypoglycemia. *Clinics in Endocrinology and Metabolism* 9(3): 461-475.

Guptaa MA, Schork NJ, Gupta AK, Kirkby S, Ellis CN. (1993). Suicidal ideation in psoriasis. *Int'l J Dermatol* 32: 188-190.

Hawton K. (1987). Assessment of suicide risk. *Brit J Psychiatry* 150: 145-153.

Hawton K, Fagg J, Marsack P. (1980). Association between epilepsy and attempted suicide. *J Neurol Neurosurg Psychiatry* 43: 168-170.

Hendler N. (1984). Depression caused by chronic pain. *J Clin Psychiatr* 45: 30-36.

Jefferys DB, Volans GN. (1983). Self poisoning in diabetic patients. *Human Toxicol* 2: 345-4833.

Kaminer Y, Robbins DR. (1983). Insulin misuse: A review of an overlooked psychiatric problem. *Psychosom* 30(1): 19-24.

Kontaxakis VP, Christodolou GN, Mavreas VG, Havaki-Kontaxaki BJ. (1988). Attempted suicide in psychiatric outpatients with concurrent physical illness. *Psychother Psychosom* 50: 201-206.

Kyvik K, Stenager EN, Svendsen A, Green A. (1994). Suicides in men with insulin-dependent diabetes mellitus. *Diabetes Care* 17: 210-212.

Mendez MF, Lanska DJ, Manon-Espaillat R, Burnstine TH. (1989). Causative factors for suicide attempts by overdose in epileptics. *Arch Neurol* 46: 1065-1068.

Nielsen B. (1994). "Prædiktorer for gentagen suicidal adfærd." PhD thesis. Odense, Denmark: Odense University Press.

Nielsen B, Wang AG, Bille-Brahe U. (1990). Attempted suicide in Denmark. IV. A five-year follow-up. *Acta Psychiatrica Scand* 81: 250-254.

Öjehagen A, Regnell G, Träskman-Bendz L. (1991). Deliberate self-poisoning: Repeaters and non-repeaters admitted to an intensive care unit. *Acta Psychiatrica Scand* 84: 266-271.

Schiffer RB. (1990). Depressive syndromes associated with diseases of the central nervous system. *Sem Neurol* 10(3): 239-246.

Simmons RG, Schilling KJ. (1974). Social and psychological rehabilitation of the diabetic transplant patient. *Kidney-Int-Suppl* 1: 152-158.

Stenager EN. (1992). Parasuicide, somatic diseases and pain. In *Suicidal behavior: The state of the art. Proceedings of the XVI. Congress of the International Association for Suicide Prevention*, K Böhme, H Wedler (eds.). Regensburg, Germany: Roderer S Verlag, pp. 869-872.

Stenager EN, Benjaminsen S. (1991). Repetition of parasuicide, psychiatric diagnosis, and treatment modalities: A one-year follow-up. In *Suicide attempts in the Nordic countries: Epidemiology and treatment*, T Bjerke, TC Stiles (eds.). Trondheim, Norway: Tapir Publishers, pp. 171-183.

Stenager EN, Jensen K. (1994). Attempted suicide: Contact to the primary health authorities. *Acta Psychiatrica Scand* 90: 109-113.

Stenager EN, Stenager E. (1992). Suicide in patients with neurological diseases: Methodological problems. Literature review. *Arch Neurol* 49: 1296-1303.

Stenager E, Knudsen L, Jensen K. (1990). Psychiatric and cognitive aspects of multiple sclerosis. *Sem Neurol* 10(3): 254-261.

Stenager EN, Stenager E, Jensen K. (1994). Depression, pain and somatic diseases: A one year follow-up study. *Psychother Psychosom* 61: 65-74.

Stenager E, Christensen LL, Jepsen I, Krarup G, Petersen P, Thygesen-Rasmussen G, Benjaminsen S. (1992). Selvmordsforsøg, diagnose og behandling. *Nord J Psychiatry* 46: 33-39.

Wedler H. (1991). Körperliche Krankheiten bei Suizidpatienten einer internistischen Abteilung. In *Körperliche Krankheit und Suizid*, H Wedler, HJ Möller (eds.). Regensburg, Germany: Roderer S Verlag, pp. 87-101.

Whitlock FA. (1986). Suicide and physical illness. In *Suicide*, A Roy (ed.). Baltimore: Williams and Wilkins, pp. 151-170.

WHO. (1986). Summary report: Working group on preventive practices in suicide and attempted suicide. York, PA: Author (JCP/PSFØ17 (S).

Wolff G. (1971). Aktuelle probleme der Hypoglykemie. *Med Welt* 22/Heft 42: 1632-1637.

Chapter 9

Adler HA, Zlot S, Hürny C, Minder C. (1989). Engel's "Psychogenic pain and the pain-prone patient": A retrospective, controlled clinical study. *Psychosomatic Med* 51: 87-101.

Andersen S, Worm-Pedersen J. (1987). The prevalence of persistent pain in a Danish population. *Pain* (Suppl) 4: 322.

Atkinson JH, Slater MA, Grant I, Patterson TL, Garfin SR. (1988). Depressed mood in chronic low back pain: Relationship with stressful life events. *Pain* 35: 47-55.

Bebbington PE. (1976). Monosymptomatic hypochondriasis, abnormal illness behaviour, and suicide. *Brit J Psychiatr* 128: 475-478.

Blumer D, Heilbronn M. (1982). Chronic pain as a variant of depressive disease: The pain prone disorder. *J Nervous and Men Dis* 170: 381-394.

Breitbart W. (1990). Cancer, pain, and suicide. *Advances in Pain Res and Ther* 16: 399-412.

Crook J, Rideout E, Browne G. (1984). The prevalence of pain complaint in a general population. *Pain* 18: 299-314.

Dufton BD. (1989). Cognitive failure and chronic pain. *Int J Psychiatry in Med* 3: 291-297.

Fishbain DA. (1995). Chronic pain and suicide. *Psychother Psychosom* 63: 54.

Fishbain DA, Goldberg M, Meagher RB, Steele R, Rosomoff H. (1986). Male and female chronic pain patients categorized by DSM-III psychiatric diagnostic criteria. *Pain* 26: 181-197.

Fishbain DA, Goldberg M, Steele Rosomoff R, Rosomoff H. (1991). Completed suicide in chronic pain. *Clin J Pain* 7: 29-36.

Hendler N. (1985). Depression caused by chronic pain. *J Clin Psychiatry* 45: 20-36.

Kotarba JA. (1983). Perceptions of death, belief systems, and the process of coping with chronic pain. *Soc Sci Med* 17: 681-689.

Livengood JM, Parris WCV. (1992). Early detection measures and triage procedures for suicide ideation in chronic pain patients. *Clin J Pain* 8(2): 164-169.

Orbach I. (1994). Dissociation, physical pain, and suicide: A hypothesis. Review article. *Suicide and Life-Threatening Behav* 24: 68-79.

Romano JM, Turner JA. (1985). Chronic pain and depression: Does the evidence support a relationship? *Psychological Bull* 97: 18-34.

Roy R, Thomas M, Matas M. (1984). Chronic pain and depression. *Compr Psychiatry* 25: 96-105.

Shneidman ES. (1993). Suicide as psychache. *J Nerv and Ment Dis* 181: 145-147.

Stenager EN, Stenager E, Jensen K. (1994). Attempted suicide, depression, and physical diseases: A 1-year follow-up study. *Psychother Psychosom* 61: 65-73.

Stenager EN, Stenager E. (1995). Chronic pain and suicide. *Psychother Psychosom* 63: 55.

Chapter 10

Bolund C. (1985a). Suicide and cancer: I. Demografic and social characteristics of cancer patients who comitted suicide in Sweden, 1973-1976. *J Phychosocial Oncol* 3(1): 17-30.

Bolund C. (1985b). Suicide and cancer II. Medical and care factors in suicides by patients in Sweden, 1973-1976. *J Phychosocial Oncol* 3(1): 31-52.

Damsbo N, Friborg S. (1989). Den suicidale patient. 1. Hyppighed og relevans af kontakten til praktiserende læger forud for suicidal handlinger. *Ugeskr Læger* 151: 826-828.

Damsbo N, Friborg S. (1989). Den suicidale patient. 2. Selvmordsmetoder, diagnoser og sociale forhold. *Ugeskr Læger* 151: 826-832.

Diekstra RFW, van Egmond M. (1989). Suicide and attempted suicide in general practice 1979-1986. *Acta Psychiatr Scand* 79: 268-275.

Lustman PJ, Amado H, Wetzel RD. (1983). Depression in diabetics: A critical appraisal. *Compr Psychiatry* 24(1): 65-74.

Lustman PJ, Griffith LS, Clouse RE, Cryer PE. (1983). Psychiatric illness in diabetes mellitus relationship to symptoms and glucose control. *J Nervous and Ment Dis* 174(12): 736-742.

Noyes R, Kathol RG. (1986). Depression and cancer. *Psychiatric Developments* 2: 77-100.

Petty F, Noyes R. (1981). Depression secondary to cancer. *Biological Psychiatry* 16(12): 1203-1220.

Rodin G, Voshart K. (1986). Depression in the medically ill: An overview. *J Psychiatry* 143(6): 696-705.

Runeson B. (1989). Mental disorder in youth suicides. *Acta Psychiatry Scand* 79: 490-497.

Sainsbury P. (1986). Depression, suicide, and suicide prevention. In *Suicide*, A Roy (ed.). Baltimore: Williams and Wilkins, pp. 73-88.

Stenager EN, Jensen K. (1994). Attempted suicide, contact to the primary health authorities. *Acta Psychiatry Scand* 90: 109-113.

Stenager EN, Koch-Henriksen N, Stenager E. (1996). Risk factors for suicide in multiple sclerosis. *Psychother Psychosom* 65: 86-90.

Index

Schizophrenia. *See* Psychiatric
   disorders
Screening tools, 93
Selection, 28-29,39
Self-destructive acts, 20
Self-poisoning, 31,56
Serotonin, 71,84
Sheriff, 2
Social implications, 98,100
Social isolation, 88
Social services, 101
Social differences, 56
Social workers, 7,103
Somatic disorders, 4-5,7,13,25-30,
   61-75,77-85
Spinal cord injuries, 41-43,49,87
   cause, 41
   prognosis, 41
   quadriplegia, 41
   suicide risk, 41-43
   symptoms, 41
Standard mortality ratio (SMR) 21-22,
   27,29,33-34,36,52-55,68,70
Statistic method, 16,26,29-30,33,42,
   52-53,69-70
Study population, 28-29
Subarachnoidal hemorrhage.
   See Cerebral stroke
Suicidal behavior, 3-5,15,25-27,
   66-67,83,88,97-99,101-103
Suicide attempt, 3-4,18-20,77-85,
   97-99,101-102
   age, 29
   definition, 77,80
   gender, 19,29,81
   methods, 80
Suicide, general aspects, 1-5
   age, 29
   black, 1
   caucasian, 1
   definition, 60,77
   ethnic minorities, 1
   gender, 3,29
   treatment, 4-5,23

Suicide methods, 1
   violent methods, 53,56
Suicide mortality rate, 1-5,44
Suicide mortality, 1-5,22,42,67
Suicide overestimation, 26
Suicide risk factors, 3-4,18-23,
   32,97-99
   age factors, 3
   biological risk factors. *See*
      5-HIAA
   psychiatric factors. *See*
      Psychiatric disorders
   social factors, 3,75
Suicide registration, 56,60,66
Suicide underestimation, 2,26,56,71
Suicide prevention, 4-5,23,97,99
Swedish Cancer Registry, 55

Tranquilizers, 15
Thrombosis. *See* Cerebral stroke
Tinnitus, 72-73
   audiology clinics, 73
   risk of suicide, 72-73

Ulcerative colitis. *See*
      Gastrointestinal disorders
United States, 1-2,28,37,68,73
UK. *See* England

Validity, 30-31,92,93

WHO, 2-3,77
   Target for Health for all, 2
   whiplash pain, 88
   working capacity, 88

Order Your Own Copy of
This Important Book for Your Personal Library!

DISEASE, PAIN, AND SUICIDAL BEHAVIOR

_____ in hardbound at $39.95 (ISBN: 0-7890-0111-X)

_____ in softbound at $19.95 (ISBN: 0-7890-0295-7)

COST OF BOOKS _____

OUTSIDE USA/CANADA/
MEXICO: ADD 20% _____

POSTAGE & HANDLING _____
(US: $3.00 for first book & $1.25
for each additional book)
Outside US: $4.75 for first book
& $1.75 for each additional book)

SUBTOTAL _____

IN CANADA: ADD 7% GST _____

STATE TAX _____
(NY, OH & MN residents, please
add appropriate local sales tax)

FINAL TOTAL _____
(If paying in Canadian funds,
convert using the current
exchange rate. UNESCO
coupons welcome.)

☐ **BILL ME LATER:** ($5 service charge will be added)
(Bill-me option is good on US/Canada/Mexico orders only;
not good to jobbers, wholesalers, or subscription agencies.)

☐ Check here if billing address is different from
shipping address and attach purchase order and
billing address information.

Signature _____

☐ **PAYMENT ENCLOSED: $** _____

☐ **PLEASE CHARGE TO MY CREDIT CARD.**

☐ Visa ☐ MasterCard ☐ AmEx ☐ Discover
☐ Diners Club
Account # _____

Exp. Date _____

Signature _____

Prices in US dollars and subject to change without notice.

NAME _____

INSTITUTION _____

ADDRESS _____

CITY _____

STATE/ZIP _____

COUNTRY _____ COUNTY (NY residents only) _____

TEL _____ FAX _____

E-MAIL_____
May we use your e-mail address for confirmations and other types of information? ☐ Yes ☐ No

Order From Your Local Bookstore or Directly From
The Haworth Press, Inc.
10 Alice Street, Binghamton, New York 13904-1580 • USA
TELEPHONE: 1-800-HAWORTH (1-800-429-6784) / Outside US/Canada: (607) 722-5857
FAX: 1-800-895-0582 / Outside US/Canada: (607) 772-6362
E-mail: getinfo@haworth.com
PLEASE PHOTOCOPY THIS FORM FOR YOUR PERSONAL USE.

BOF96